THE HANDB
FOR
COMMUNITY
CARE
ASSISTANTS
AND SUPPORT WORKERS

Edited by Stuart Darby and Sue Benson

A Care Concern Publication

First published in 1995 by
Hawker Publications Ltd
13 Park House
140 Battersea Park Road
London SW11 4NB

British Library Cataloguing in Publication Data

A catalogue record for this book is available
from the British Library

ISBN 1 874790 18 3

Designed by
Richard Souper

Phototypeset by
Hawker Publications

Printed and bound in Great Britain by
Butler and Tanner, Frome, Somerset

*One of the illustrations in Chapter 14 is redrawn from How to Save a Life by Alan Maryon Davies
and Jenny Rogers, BBC Books. Other illustrations by Eve Morris.*

Other titles in this series:
Handbook for Care Assistants – A Practical Guide to Caring for Elderly People
Fourth Edition 1995. ISBN 1 874790 19 1
The Care Assistant's Guide to Working With Elderly Mentally Infirm People
Second Edition 1994. ISBN 1 874790 15 9
A Practical Guide to Working with People With Learning Disabilities
Second Edition 1994. ISBN 1 874790 12 4
The Handbook for Hospital Care Assistants and Support Workers
1993. ISBN 1 874790 10 8

Contents

Contributors

June Andrews RMN RGN MA is secretary to the Scottish Board of the Royal College of Nursing. Her clinical experience has been in nursing elderly and elderly mentally ill people.

Rose Ashbee is manager of the Royal National Institute for the Blind's Westcliff House, Westgate on Sea, Kent. She began her career as a care assistant with RNIB, and has trained in social work and communication with the deaf-blind.

Veronica Beasley Dip COT has worked as an occupational therapist in psychiatry and general medicine. For the last ten years, she has worked for the London Borough of Islington as a community occupational therapist.

Lesley Bell is executive director of the joint initiative for community care, chair of the joint advisory group of domiciliary care associations, and a non-executive director of a community health trust.

Sue Benson BA RGN is an experienced practising nurse and specialist editor of health care educational projects.

Karen Bryan PhD BSc MCSLT is a lecturer in acquired communication disorders at the National Hospitals College of Speech Sciences. She is currently involved in developing a communication training programme for care assistants.

Hilary Brown MSc is senior lecturer in learning disabilities at the Tizard Centre, University of Kent. She has experience of working in residential services and as a trainer, and has devised training exercises and manuals. She is currently involved in research and policy concerning abuse of vulnerable adults.

Jo Carroll RGN DipHV has worked as a ward sister in acute care of older people and is now employed as a health visitor in Tower Hamlets.

Jill Cowley RGN NDN CDT PN Cert is an experienced district nurse, and is currently working as a senior nurse in general practice in Gainsborough, Lincolnshire.

Alan Crump BSc(Hons)Nursing RGN RMN, is a charge nurse in the Nursing Development Unit, Seacroft Hospital, Leeds, and an executive member of the Royal College of Nursing membership group, *Focus: on older people nursing and mental health*.

Liz Day MA (Gerontology) BA RGN NDN HV PGCEA is a senior lecturer at Croydon College. Her special interests include ageing, health promotion and social sciences. She worked as a specialist health visitor with older people and people with disabilities in a social work team.

Stuart Darby BA RGN RMN RHV DPSN is the head of community nursing development team, Camden and Islington Community Health Services NHS Trust. He has worked as a health visitor, and clinical nurse specialist in mental health care of older people. He is currently chair of the RCN group *Focus: on older people, nursing and mental health*.

Valerie Good BSc CQSW DMS Cert Ed. has worked extensively with older people with mental health problems, both as a practitioner and a manager. She is currently involved in strategic planning and service development.

Louise Hembrough BA RGN RHV has worked as a senior nurse at Atkinson Morley's Hospital, Wimbledon, having completed a post graduate diploma in community nursing. She is now practising as a health visitor in Tower Hamlets.

Judith Hodgkinson BA DipAdEd worked for several years with The Centre for Policy on Ageing to improve residential care practice, and advised on resources for adult learning and training with the Health Education Authority. She now manages a domiciliary respite service for carers and people with dementia, for Islington Crossroads Care Attendant Scheme.

Marion Judd MSc MCSP MNZSP has worked as a community physiotherapist and is currently employed as a clinical audit officer with Camden and Islington Community Health Services NHS Trust.

Mansour Olawale Jumaa MSc BA DipNEd PGdip Hon Psych RN RNT is the director of continuing education and NVQ co-ordinator at the North London College of Health Studies, and associate colleague of Middlesex University.

Tim Martin RNN BSc Hons has worked in rehabilitation and resettlement for eight years as a senior nurse and is currently the manager of a community mental health unit in Salford.

Jane Maxim PhD MA DipCST MCSLT is a senior lecturer at the National Hospitals College of Speech Sciences. She is a speech therapist whose research area is language change in dementia, and she works with elderly stroke patients.

Lyn Meehan BSc RGN Dip Nursing (Lond) NDN Cert Ed RNT. She has previously worked as a district nurse and is now director of Community Nursing Studies at Bloomsbury and Islington College of Nursing and Midwifery. She is undertaking a Masters degree in Gerontology at Kings College, London.

Eric Midwinter is a past director of the Centre for Policy on Ageing. Now "retired" he works as consultant to projects in a wide variety of fields, including old age and education.

Judith Roberts RGN RSCN Cert Health Ed is a lecturer at Wirral Metropolitan College, and acts as joint co-ordinator of Wirral Social Care Assessment Centre, a joint partnership between Wirral Metropolitan College and Wirral Social Services.

Alison Robertson RGN RSCN PGdipHV is a cystic fibrosis home care nurse at the Royal Brompton Hospital. She previously worked as a paediatric community nurse at the Children's Hospital, Lewisham.

Vicky Robinson is a clinical nurse manager. She currently manages a palliative care team attached to UCH/Middlesex hospitals. She has extensive experience in both practical care and counselling people with terminal illness.

Sally Shulman BPharm MRPharmS is the principal pharmacist working for Camden and Islington Community Health Services NHS Trust. Previously she worked for 11 years in a pharmacy in North West London.

Helen White RGN RHV is continence adviser for Disability North at the Dene Centre, Newcastle upon Tyne Council for the Disabled.

Jennie Williams RGN PG Dip in District Nursing has worked as a ward sister in acute care of older people and as a clinical nurse teacher. More recently, she has worked as a district nurse and Professional Development Nurse for community nurses working with adults and older people in Camden and Islington Community Health Services NHS Trust.

Introduction

This book provides care assistants with the necessary knowledge and skills to provide high standards of care to people in their own homes and elsewhere in the community.

The Community Care Act 1990, implemented in April 1993, has reaffirmed that people who choose to remain at home must be offered a range of choices and services. These must be planned, organised and delivered in partnership with them. In addition, earlier hospital discharges and an increase in high technology care at home, means that increased support and help may be required in the home where this may once have been provided in a hospital setting.

A broad approach has been taken to ensure that each chapter meets the needs of the large number of care assistants employed by public, voluntary and independent agencies. Therefore, we have decided to use the term *care assistant* throughout the book and *qualified member of staff* to denote a more senior person taking overall responsibility. We do not suggest that one person's role is more important than another. We believe that every person providing care must share the same values of respecting client independence and dignity in carrying out their duties to the highest possible standards.

Throughout the book we acknowledge both the contribution and the needs of the many carers who work voluntarily or care for loved ones, friends and relatives at home.

The environment and "community" in which people live must be considered. Consequently, we have included chapters that consider health and wellbeing from "cradle to grave". We have included chapters on supporting parents and guardians to ensure healthy child development, and chapters that consider the provision of services which will identify client needs, promote wellbeing and anticipate and prevent further problems, as well as chapters on providing practical care and attention to people with long term progressive and terminal illnesses.

The book also meets the needs of care assistants working within other care settings who may be required to visit a client at home. This may be before admission, discharge or during an episode of respite care. We believe that encouraging good collaboration between a range of service providers is essential to ensuring continuity of care.

Finally, we have used the National Vocational Qualifications and Scottish Vocational Qualifications in Care as a framework for each topic. We have purposely limited our coverage of each subject to essential units, and while we have listed only Level 2 Core, Direct Care and Domiciliary Support units at the end of each chapter, the full range of units covered can be seen in the charts on pages 184-186. We hope that this approach will provide a focus for the many different forms of training we think care assistants should be offered, and that they will find the book a useful resource to help them achieve these practical, skill-based qualifications.

Stuart Darby and Sue Benson

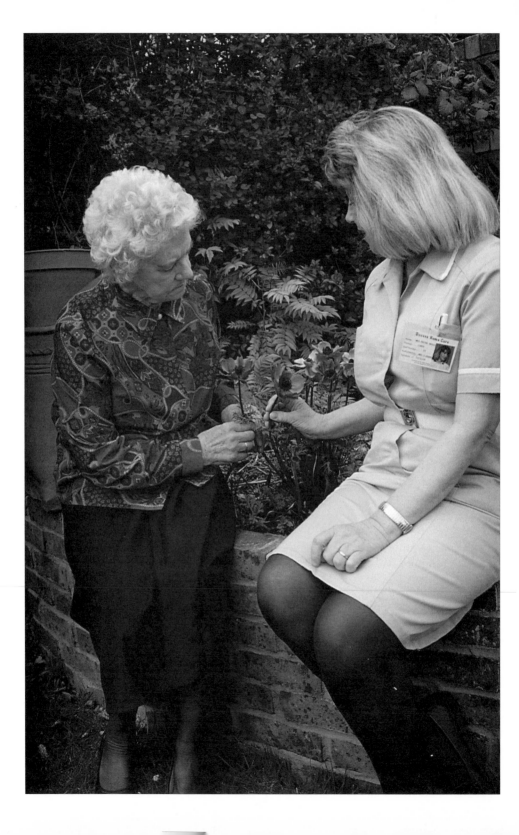

CHAPTER 1

Care in the community

Stuart Darby and Lyn Meehan

• What is a community? • How can the community care? • Community care legislation • Your role as a care assistant • Ensuring quality services

Home is a very important place. We all have different homes. These might be houses, flats, hostels, residential or nursing homes. Some people may have a home of a temporary nature such as a hostel or bed and breakfast accommodation. Other people may have no home at all and be "homeless". "Home" is therefore something personal and special to each of us. The way that we decorate, the furniture, the garden and our families or partners are a very large part of our lives.

Enabling people stay in their own homes is an essential contribution to their physical, social and mental health and wellbeing.

Care in the community involves looking after people in their own homes. New laws have shifted health and social care away from large long-stay hospitals to home care services that can be arranged though a variety of agencies. The aim is to promote a greater choice of options for people wishing to stay at home. We need a knowledge and understanding of community boundaries, where the community starts and ends. We also need a knowledge of community components: how it is made up, who lives there and activities that take place, in order to provide effective and efficient services.

What is a community?

Defining "the community" is difficult. It means different things to different people. It can be more than just a place in which people live. We can see this when we look at terms such as "European Economic Community" (now known as the European Union – EU) or "community spirit". A residential or a geographical area in which people live and feel that they belong, can be defined as a community. In addition some people may work in one community while living in another. Industrial organisations, schools, large companies and hospitals may also be described as communities. This may lead to different behaviour as a work role can be very different from a social role. For example, a working mother may have one role in the workplace and another at home, with her partner and children.

Defining the community

We use two types of information to define communities. Firstly, facts that can be counted. These include Census statistics on the number and age of people, their ethnic origin, types of housing and the number of people employed. Secondly we can include subjective information, such as an individual's perceptions, opinions and feelings about where they live and whether they feel safe, comfortable and happy.

A community therefore is made up of a whole range of factors. Care in the community includes providing services to people of all ages. Some people will be fit and healthy. Others may require short episodes of care for acute illness, or care through a long-term and progressive illness that may lead eventually to death.

How can a community care?

The idea of community care is both vague and diverse. It has largely come to mean either the provision of care by domiciliary services or a notion of care given by the community and society. Domiciliary services are important and provide care which a family is unable to give. Nevertheless, the support of family and friends is important to the complete health and wellbeing of an individual.

You might like to consider a description of community care as it might appear to:

• a carer
• an older or disabled person
• a politician
• a health or social care provider such as yourself.

What are the main conflicts between these different people?

Community Care Legislation

The main legislation that influences the way community care is provided includes:

1. The Chronically Sick and Disabled Persons Act 1970
2. The NHS and Community Care Act 1990
3. The Children Act 1989

The Chronically Sick and Disabled Persons Act 1970
The Chronically Sick and Disabled

Persons Act was intended to become a charter for people with a disability. Although there have been more recent amendments, the major provisions remain the same.

Mandatory arrangements should be in place for each local authority to establish the number of people with a disability in their area and to find out their needs. There is no obligation on the disabled person to register with the local authority. Since there is no standard agreement on what "disability" actually means, local authorities have their own definitions, often with great variation between them. Essentially, the Acts give power to enable a disabled person to:

• obtain practical help in the home
• obtain recreational facilities and travelling to get to them
• adapt their home to secure greater safety, comfort and convenience
• obtain meals in the home or elsewhere
• obtain a telephone and any equipment needed to use this.

Local authorities were also empowered to ensure that access is made available to facilities such as public toilets. Orange badge labels which give parking concessions are issued for display in motor vehicles. Some local authorities may also provide special housing.

Many people with disabilities are not sick. They are living with impairments which handicap them to a greater or lesser extent, depending on the opportunities available to them. They need a range of support from statutory and voluntary agencies. They need someone to help with practical everyday tasks such as shopping and cooking. They may need adaptations to their home, financial support or help to find suitable employment. They may need help with transport and mobility. They will need general health care and may need specialist advice, care and therapy.

Community care: How it all fits together

ROLE OF THE CARE ASSISTANT
- Working with individuals to provide practical help and care
- Working with families and carers to support them
- Working with the wider comunity to encourage good health and wellbeing
- Working with other services to ensure a coordinated approach to care

WHAT IS A COMMUNITY?
- A place in which people live or work
- A feeling of belonging to particular group of individuals
- An area defined by geography
- An area defined for organisational and administrative boundaries
- Components, how it is made up, who lives there and activities or incident that take place within it

FACTORS AFFECTING CARE IN THE COMMUNITY
- Health care and social care
- Health and wellbeing of individuals
- Employment
- Education
- Housing and environment
- Personal disability
- Finance and income
- History of the area
- 'Social' climate, crime and vandalism
- Transport
- Leisure and recreational activities

HOW DOES THE COMMUNITY CARE?
- Support from carers, families and others
- Health services, nurses, GPs, hospitals and others
- Local authorities, housing, waste disposal and emergency services
- Social services
- Voluntary and independent sector services

LEGISLATION
- The Chronically Sick and Disabled Persons Act 1970
- The NHS and Commmunity Care Act 1990.
- The Children Act 1989
- Local Council Tax

Chapter 9 considers some issues that you may need to consider when providing care to a person with a disability.

The NHS and Community Care Act 1990

The NHS and Community Care Act aims to enable people to live as independently as possible in their own homes or in a homely setting in the community. This includes those with long term physical and mental illness or disability who could not remain at home without increased help and support. The Act also promotes the use of independent agencies to encourage a wider range of choices in services to be made available. To achieve this, each local authority is responsible for employing care managers. The care manager's role is to ensure that a good assessment of client and carer needs (what people want, rather than what is traditionally available) takes place. He or she is responsible for coordinating and meeting care needs in consultation with clients, carers and a range of other care providers. As a care assistant you may be asked to contribute to community living assessments. You will have a close working relationship with clients and carers and this will enable you to add information that could improve their care.

The Children Act 1989

The Children Act draws together all the relevant laws and recommends that wherever possible, children should be cared for within their own families. If they are in danger, they should be kept safe and protected, perhaps through court action. They should always be asked about their wishes and be kept informed about what happens to them.

Children may be referred to as "in need" meaning that their normal health and development may be at risk if special services are not arranged for them. There must be specialist community workers in each area to advise on children in need. These specialists are responsible for working closely with parents, guardians, social services, health and local authority departments. They must ensure that children in need are assessed and referred to agencies that will help ensure a healthy physical and emotional childhood and development.

Your role as a care assistant

Your role will include four main duties:
1. Working with individuals to provide practical help and care.
2. Working with families and carers to support them.
3. Working with the wider community to encourage good health and wellbeing.
4. Working with other caring services to ensure a coordinated approach.
As a care assistant you can contribute to the work of other staff in meeting the requirements of the Community Care Act and The Children Act. You will need to work closely and under supervision, with clients, children, carers and parents. Your work will include enhancing their knowledge and understanding of their rights. It will include listening to your clients and taking account of their wishes and feelings where appropriate.

You may be asked to cooperate and collaborate with other agencies, such as education departments. If you contribute to a community living assessment or to a report on a child and their family, always report the facts of what you have seen and heard. If you are concerned about a client always discuss this with a qualified member of staff. Remember that all information about another person must be held in strict confidence.

Working with individuals

Your care to an individual client is clearly going to be the aspect that you concentrate upon most. However, the whole family, and particularly people who care for others at home, are also important. Developing a trusting relationship is dependent upon your skills in approaching clients, and your behaviour.

If you are contributing to assessments, care plans or giving care, people need to feel safe, reassured and comfortable in the knowledge that you will respect their individual privacy (see chapter 15). Understanding and explaining your own role and the role of different agencies will help clients to understand why you are there and what activity you can carry out. If you, the client and/or their carer understand and have clearly stated objectives, you can work together. This is important to achieve both short and long term goals.

Remember that you will be a guest in someone's home. Your visits should always be planned and pre-arranged. Make certain that you have adequate time and regular contact to build up reliable relationships. Confidentiality is essential. Clients need to be sure that any information or knowledge that you have about them will only be used for their own benefit and will not be shared with other people.

Listening to what people say and asking appropriate questions is important so that clients feel that their needs and wants are respected and considered. To actively listen you need to be free from distractions, comfortably close to the person and ready to acknowledge their personal and cultural needs. (See chapter 5, Talking and listening.) You should never judge another person's lifestyle simply because it does not fit in with your own ideas or beliefs.

The impact of sickness and disability on the individual and people close to them

When people are ill, they often have an altered mental image of themselves. They may feel that their personal strengths and weaknesses are changed. They may feel left out of decision making and social functions. There is also a danger that they do not feel themselves a valued part of their family. This can also occur when people have experienced a physical change to their body, such as a scar, a loss of limb or function of limb, or weight loss. Helping people to adapt and accept these changes can take a long time.

People who are ill may also experience a change in their role. Some will have been wage earners and responsible for other dependent partners or children. Families often take over responsibilities and everyday challenges. This can lead to a sense of loss similar to bereavement or loss of employment. It is important to recognise these tensions and conflicts as they can also occur between care workers and others who provide care at home.

Episodes of care

Unlike care in residential or nursing homes, care to people in their own homes is usually carried out in episodes. Episodes of care may relate to a person's illness or disability. A person who is discharged from hospital may only require care and visits for a few weeks. Other people may come to your attention if they have an illness that improves, but they then require help again. Finally, some people will need long term care over a period of months and sometimes years. Your role is equally important whatever period or frequency you visit. Ensuring that people are safe and able to be independent on leaving the home or ending an episode of care is one of most important features of providing care in the community.

Different skills

You will need a range of skills to provide care in the community. You will meet many different people, all of whom will require different types of care. Some people may be physically fit, healthy and require health education and advice. Others will have actual problems or potential problems because of their lifestyle.

Different care settings

Working in the community can mean providing care in a variety of settings. This may be in a person's own home, residential or nursing home. It may mean providing care in a social setting such as a day care centre or luncheon club. Many areas also have special meetings for carers or those with a particular problem, such as Stroke Clubs or Alzheimer's Disease Society Meetings. You may also need to carry out care in hostels or accommodation for those people who are homeless.

Families and carers

The term carer is used to describe people undertaking many different tasks in differing situations. These can range from shopping, to providing twenty-four hour care. Most carers are in their middle years and are looking after parents. There are greater numbers of female than male carers, and men are less likely to be caring for another person outside their own home. In recent years carer groups and organisations have campaigned for their needs to be recognised and valued. This is an important part of providing care. Your skills need to include listening to carers and respecting their knowledge about the condition and care of the person they look after. You also need to encourage them to pay attention to their own physical and emotional needs.

The wider community

The broader community also needs to be considered. The people who live in an area contribute to its "social climate". They can also be helped to take responsibility for a safe and healthy environment. For example, many areas operate environmental health schemes where residents can quickly report things like poor street lighting or broken paving slabs. These can then be acted upon and the health and safety of residents protected.

Primary preventive care and early discovery of problems

This includes giving health education, advice and information based on our knowledge of what causes ill health and disease. Examples may include people who want to take more exercise, choose a healthier diet, give up smoking or require holiday vaccinations in order for them to remain well. Screening for physical and mental health problems (often known as secondary preventive care) is included in this range of duties. This enables potential health problems to be identified and dealt with before the onset of further damage. Examples of this include child development screening, checking adults who may be at risk from coronary heart disease or certain cancers, and assessing people over the age of 75 years (see chapter 7).

Supportive and health maintaining care

This type of care aims to prevent the deterioration of an established condition or to promote rehabilitation and maintain a certain level of quality of life. People who are dying can still have an improved quality of life if they can undertake the things that they want to do and be free from pain. Families with a child with learning difficulties can be helped by reducing problems and disruption to their lives. They need help to encourage them to reach their potential, support through emotional crises, and practical help and information.

Working with groups

Many community workers also provide services and help to groups of people who share common needs. A good example is the needs of carers. "Group work" can take many forms. Examples include health education courses, teaching at Stroke Clubs and participating in citizens advice meetings to provide information on how to access health and social services. Working with groups of people demands different skills, but it is just as important as one-to-one care. People can gain a lot of strength from sharing problems and receiving help and information on how to overcome them.

Environmental factors that affect health and wellbeing

The environment that a person lives in can greatly influence their physical, emotional and social well being. You might like to think about the examples given below:

Environment

• What type of housing is available and is it suitable to a person's needs?
• Is there access to parks, leisure centres, libraries and recreational activities?
• Is there a high crime rate, excessive vandalism or a large drug or alcohol dependency problem in the area?

Support and caring services

• Is it a "close knit" community?
• Do people have a network of support from neighbours, friends or relatives?
• Are religious, cultural and community groups available?
• Are GPs nearby?

- Can social service departments be accessed easily?
- Is there a local hospital that is easy to reach?

Employment
- Are there high levels of unemployment?
- Has industry closed down or moved away, leaving people with skills but no work?
- Do people have enough money to meet their needs?

Local facilities
- How close are shops and other facilities?
- Is there a launderette or place for people to wash their clothes?
- How close is the nearest post office for people who need to collect benefits?
- Is the transport system good and can people easily get around?

You can see from this list that you need to think about a whole range of issues when considering the health and wellbeing of an individual, as well as providing care to them at home.

Coordinating services

Many different agencies provide health and social care in the community. The chart on page 11 illustrates some services that contribute to health and wellbeing, including public health, social and local authority, and voluntary and independent sector services.

Your work in collaboration with other agencies is essential if coordinated and effective care is to be offered and carried out. Clients and their carers need to be fully involved in planning and agreeing how their needs can be met. They need to be offered a range of options and choices. Active partnership and participation will encourage independence and prevent people from losing their dignity. Shared goals and objectives may be short-term or long-term, but they should always be achievable, realistic, and reviewed and changed as required.

One of the key issues affecting community care is the channelling of funds away from traditional health and social care services to independent and voluntary agencies. It is hoped that this "market" approach will encourage competition between service providers and provide a greater range and choice of services. In theory, people will be able to "shop around", in much the same way that we choose what we buy from different shops or companies.

Ensuring quality services

Setting standards and measuring quality through audit is a method of ensuring that community care is provided at the highest possible level. Standards may include statements, for example, on the hours that services are provided and when clients can expect a visit. They can also refer to policies and procedures, such as what treatment or care activity to expect. Standards are then measured or audited to make certain that these expectations are being met and how well they are being met.

What is a standard?

A standard is a statement of care that defines what activity will be carried out, where it will be undertaken and who will undertake it. A standard is usually made up of three components. The structure is the part of the standard that states where the service will be provided, what equipment may be used and who will provide the service. The process refers to what care activities will be carried out and how they will be performed. This part of the statement looks at what has been done, how well it was done and what the effect has been.

One example might include giving pain

relieving medicines to a client at home. The structure would include when you would visit, what documentation you would complete and any specific equipment or tools you might use. The process would include the medicines you give and the way in which they are given. The outcome would be to ensure that clients receive the correct medicine and dose at the right time. It would also include the client's satisfaction with the way in which the medicines were given and the amount of pain relief achieved.

Measuring standards

Measuring or auditing these components may highlight a need to change some or all of the standard. Taking the example of medicine again, you might need to change the time of giving a dose, or its strength, or the client and carer may feel that a liquid rather than a tablet would be more acceptable.

Although this is a simple example, standards exist at all levels of service delivery and can be measured by a range of people. "Purchasers", those people who buy services on behalf of clients, will be looking to ensure that the best quality services are delivered, that clients are happy with the service and that the best value for money is being achieved. "Providers", the people for whom you work, will want to ensure that clients receive a service that is acceptable, safe, causes them no harm, and that the highest professional standards are delivered efficiently and effectively.

Measuring standards involves making sure that clients and carers are happy with the service and that organisations and staff are carrying out their duties to provide the best possible service. The main aim is to ensure that clients and their carers have the opportunity to comment on services so that they can be changed to best meet their needs. A knowledge of how people can complain about a service, and ensuring that complaints are heard and acted upon, are all part of maintaining quality standards.

Further Reading
Department of Health/Royal College of Nursing (1992) *The Children Act 1989. What every nurse, health visitor and midwife needs to know.* Health Publications Unit, Heywood. Lancashire.
Department of Health/Royal College of Nursing (1993) *Community Care. What hospital nurses and community nurses need to know.* Health Publications Unit, Heywood. Lancashire.

NVQ Level 2 & 3 Core Units
O Promote equality for all individuals
U4 Contribute to the health, safety and security of individuals and their environment.
U5 Obtain, transmit and store information relating to the delivery of a care service.

Level 2 Core Unit
W2 Contribute to the ongoing support of clients and others significant to them.

Level 2 Domiciliary support
W8 Enable clients to maintain contacts in potentially isolating situations.

Level 3 Core Unit
Y2 Enable clients to make use of available services and information.

CHAPTER 2

Safeguards, rights and legal obligations

Lesley Bell

• The rights of the individual • Relevant legislation • Manual handling operations regulations • Important areas of good practice • Security in the home

Being aware of relevant legislation that safeguards individual rights is an important part of providing care to people living in their own homes. You do not need detailed knowledge, but you should be aware of the broad areas of your work covered by legislation. Knowing when to seek the advice of your first line manager and being aware of guidance and training provided by your employing organisation is essential to providing safe and effective care.

Most of the current legislation has been passed in relation to the work place rather than in private homes. The legislation has been passed to protect in different ways, all those people receiving care, the person providing care (the care assistant), and your employing authority.

There are however particular implications and areas of good practice that need to be considered when working in someone's home. If you are self employed, you may be personally responsible for meeting the requirements of relevant legislation. All care staff should have insurance that covers you for any accidents or mistakes that you may make. "Personal indemnity" is usually included if you belong to a trade union or professional body.

Rights of the individual

It is worth remembering that each of us possesses personal rights. The rights listed below are particularly important to the requirements of legislation in practice:

• To independence
• To privacy
• To dignity and respect
• To make their own decisions
• To retain their personal lifestyle
• To contribute to decisions concerning their personal care
• To be informed
• To take risks
• Not to be discriminated against.

Relevant legislation

The relevant and most important legislation is listed below:
• The Health and Safety at Work Act 1974
• Environmental Protection Act 1990
• Sex Discrimination Act 1975
• Race Relations Act 1976
• Access to Health Records Act 1990
• Data Protection Act 1984
• Personal Information Act 1989
• Control of Substances Hazardous to Health Act (COSHH) 1990
• NHS and Community Care Act 1990

• Food Safety Act 1990
• Manual Handling Regulations 1992

This chapter looks briefly at each of these pieces of legislation. You will find that individual chapters in the book also refer to these Acts and may provide more detail where appropriate.

The Health and Safety at Work Act 1994

This is arguably the most important Act. By promoting safe working environments and practice, this Act aims to prevent accidents, protect employees from the danger of fire and preserve health. The legislation protects the health and safety of the person receiving care and the people providing care.

All employing authorities have a duty to observe the requirements of the Act and to ensure that they are being carried out. This will include inspecting work premises to identify and correct potential health and safety hazards. Because your work will be undertaken in people's own homes, your employing organisation will have no authority or power to correct the hazard against the wishes of the person. To do so would be an infringement of their personal rights.

The following list outlines some of the responsibilities of employing authorities under the Act:

• Provide and maintain equipment and systems of work that are safe and without risk to health.
• Ensure arrangements for handling, storing and transporting articles and substances are safe and without risk to health.
• Provide and maintain instructions, training and supervision as necessary to ensure the health and safety at work of employees.
• Clarify those tasks which should not be undertaken because of the risks to safety.

Hazards in the home

You also have a responsibility under the Health and Safety at Work Act to report any problems and ensure that appropriate action is taken. If you do identify any potential hazards in your client's home you should discuss these with your line manager. Clients may need help to make their environment safe, such as replacing a light bulb or making minor changes so that you can manoeuvre around the home safely. The following list highlights some main issues:

• Electrical hazards – faulty wiring, trailing flexes, overloaded electricity sockets and frayed cables.
• Fires – unprotected open fires, free standing electric, paraffin or gas fires, clothes drying in front of a naked flame.
• Carpets – frayed or worn carpets and loose mats (particularly on stairs).
• Kitchen – faulty appliances, leaking gas taps, bad wiring, out of date and mouldy food.
• General – poorly lit stairs and slippery floors.

Dirty and infested homes

On occasions you may be asked to care for a client who has a very dirty or infested home. It is important not to be judgemental, as there are many reasons why people are unable to maintain standards of hygiene and cleanliness. Some people may have mental health needs while others may not be physically able to clean. Such situations arise for many reasons and may be caused by:

• Years of neglect and lack of cleanliness
• Hoarding goods, particularly rubbish, old newspapers, bottles.
• Keeping large number of pets and being unable to look after them.

Inevitably, homes can become infested with vermin such as rats, cockroaches and lice. There are usually special teams who have protective clothing and equipment to clear homes that are dirty and infested.

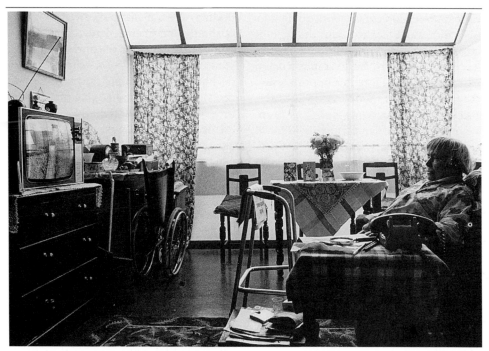

Under the Community Care Act, people who need help to stay in their own homes should have their needs assessed and have as much choice as possible in the way care is provided.

The Environmental Protection Act 1990

Under this Act, if you are responsible for producing, carrying, keeping or disposing of "waste" as part of your duties, you must ensure that this is carried out safely. Care assistants are often involved in the disposal of "clinical waste". This may include incontinence pads, needles and syringes or other sharps and equipment used to treat a client. Each employer must have policies and guidelines in place for ensuring the most appropriate and safe disposal of clinical waste. Many organisations have special coloured and marked bags or boxes. These must always be used. This protects the environment and other people who may be handling the waste bags.

Sex Discrimination Act 1975 and Race Relations Act 1976

These two Acts make it unlawful to discriminate against anyone because of their gender or race. This includes clients dis-

criminating against you as a care assistant. All employing authorities should offer written information and training on policies relating to equal opportunities (see chapter 3).

Race

Clearly, it is rarely possible to "match" care assistants to clients. It is important therefore that you have a knowledge of each client's cultural or religious background. This will help to ensure that all care will meet individual needs and will not cause offence.

Providing care to people from black and ethnic minority communities is also covered in chapter 4. This will help you to consider each person's individual rights in relation to their beliefs and values.

Gender

We all have stereotypes about men and women. Take care not to let them shape your attitudes and expectations about people's individual lifestyles and the type of activities you carry out. Sex discrimination has occurred where, for example, women may be given fewer career opportunities, they are paid less money or do not have the same employment rights as men. Women are also the main providers of unpaid care to people at home. Many people believe that society discriminates against women as this prevents them from doing what they want to do or from earning an income.

Equal opportunities can also include the avoidance of discrimination against people because of a disability or their sexual orientation.

Access to Health Records Act 1990 and Data Protection Act 1984

Everyone has a right to know what personal information and data is recorded and kept about them. The Access to Records Act generally refers to information kept in manual records such as case notes and care plans. The Data Protection Act is extended to information held on computers.

The Access to Health Records Act 1990 gives clients the right of access to their manually held records written after 1st November 1991. The term "health record" includes all manually held records made by or on behalf of a health professional. There is no advantage in keeping private records as clients can also have access to these.

Clients or any individual authorised by them, can make an application to see their records, by whoever holds them, at that time. In the case of a child, a parent or guardian may apply. An application can also be made after the death of a client by their personal representative, or a person who may have claim, for example, in the case of a disputed will.

In certain rare circumstances a GP may decline access if disclosure is, in the view of the doctor, likely to cause harm to the client's physical or mental condition. Where the holder of a health record declines access, the applicant may apply to the County Court or High Court for an order enforcing their rights of access.

It is important therefore that all notes are objective and accurate. Corrections can be made to records if they are deemed to be incomplete or incorrect. Any correction should not obscure the original entry.

Under the Data Protection Act 1984, clients are also entitled to apply for access to any personal information held on computer. The information must have been obtained fairly and lawfully. Only data that is essential and accurate should be kept on record. It is an offence to reveal confidential information from a computer to someone who is not authorised to see it. Those who wish to see their personal computer records are required to pay a fee and complete the appropriate form. Clients have the right to have information erased or corrected in a similar way to the Access to Health Records Act.

It is always good practice to share notes with clients and carers. Do remember that these are personal and confidential to them. Wherever possible seek the agreement of clients before making records of any kind. This protects their right to privacy and ensures that they can control and actively participate in their own care. Many care plans now have a space for the client or carer to sign. This will show that they agree with what has been planned or what care has been carried out.

Control of Substances Hazardous to Health Act 1988 (COSHH)

This Act seeks to safeguard those people who may be at risk if exposed to harmful or hazardous substances. Examples include cleaning and decorating materials and pest control materials. It can also include substances such as mercury in thermometers.

Your employing organisation will have a duty to comply with the regulations and not to expose you to undue risk. There will usually be a procedure book detailing the action that you should take with hazardous substances.

All hazardous substances are marked with an orange or red box with a black cross and the words:

• Corrosive

• Very Toxic

• Toxic

• Harmful Irritant

It is very important that you always follow the instructions relating to the storage and handling of these substances. Any protective clothing or equipment, such as eye goggles or gloves must be used where specified. An example in practice includes the breakage of a thermometer, and the way in which you mop up spilt mercury and dispose of it.

The most effective way to ensure that the requirements of the Act are met, is to use safe products that are not labelled in the way described above. There are many products easily available, which do not contain dangerous chemicals, yet undertake the same job just as effectively. These should always be used instead of more dangerous substances.

You should always encourage clients to use or buy safe products and store them in a safe place. However, the final decision on what to purchase is theirs.

NHS and Community Care Act 1990

This Act provides the framework for much of the work that you will be undertaking. It is also discussed in chapter 1.

The main requirements are that people who need a significant amount of help to remain living in their own homes, should have their care needs assessed. Social Service Departments must designate a specific person known as a care manager. An assessment and care plan, designed in partnership with the client, carer and other agencies must be drawn up and agreed. A range of public, voluntary and independent sector services can be commissioned to provide care. This ensures that people have the maximum amount of choice to stay at home and in the way that care is provided.

You should always be aware of care plans for each person. Ideally, each client will have their own copy. See also chapter 15 on practical care in the home. This will tell you what types of activity are planned and who will be undertaking them. Collaborative and coordinated work with other community care agencies is a key aim of the Act.

Complaints

One other main requirement of the Act is that formal complaints procedures should be in place and widely publicised. You will need to be familiar with the complaints procedure for your employing authority so that you can bring this to the attention of clients and their carers. Do try to think of complaints as a useful way of changing and adapting services to improve them. Nobody likes to think that the care that they give is poor. Often complaints are a symptom of the way in which services are organised rather than about individual people themselves.

The Food Safety Act 1990

This Act relates to food hygiene and the preparation and provision of food. Although the Act refers to designated work places, you may be involved in preparing food for clients and the following basic procedures should always be observed:

• Always wash your hands before handling food and after using the toilet.

• Ensure that cuts and sores are covered with a clean waterproof dressing.
• Keep clean and wear clean clothing.
• Keep hands off food as far as possible.
• Prepare raw and cooked foods on separate work surfaces or make sure that utensils are cleaned between preparing raw and cooked food.
• Keep food covered and either refrigerated or very hot.
• Ensure waste food is disposed of properly.
• Keep the lid on the dustbin and wash hands after use.
• Keep all equipment and surfaces clean.
• Do not smoke where food is prepared.
• Never cough or sneeze over food.

Manual handling regulations 1992
Practical lifting and handling of clients is covered in chapter 17. The regulations however also apply to lifting other equipment and objects as part of your duties. Where there is the risk of injury, every effort should be taken to redesign or avoid the task so that injury is reduced or removed. For example, it may be possible to show a person how to move themselves, or to arrange for bath aids, equipment or a portable hoist to be installed.

All employing authorities must provide training and guidance on manual handling and assess the likely risks of injury in every situation. Clearly, each client and their home will be different and therefore a qualified member of staff or person skilled in lifting and handling can advise. Physiotherapists and occupational therapists are employed by community health and local authority departments who can also help with this.

Money and gifts

Handling other people's money
Your duties may include collecting pensions, paying bills and doing the shopping for clients that you care for. Great care should be taken when handling money. Try to keep bills and receipts when spending clients' money so that you can present these to the person concerned. You should ensure that your client knows exactly how much money you have taken and how much change has been returned. Always keep your own money separate from your client's.

Collecting pensions should only be undertaken if you are authorised by your employer. Your client must also give permission and sign the appropriate slip.

You should always resist getting involved with a person's finances such as withdrawing money from a bank or building society. These activities are more appropriately undertaken by a relative or person given legal powers.

Gifts
The Prevention of Corruption Acts, 1906 and 1916 make it an offence for any employee to accept gifts that may induce them to refrain from doing anything in their official capacity or to show favour or disfavour to any person. This includes gifts from clients and manufacturers or organisations.

It is natural for some clients to want to give gifts to show their gratitude, particularly at Christmas or birthday time. Most employing organisations will have a written policy on accepting gifts, and some may even allow small infrequent gifts such as soap, toiletries, chocolate or house plants. You should however try to discourage this. Sharing a cake and having a cup of coffee in the course of your working visits would be a better way of receiving praise or celebrating a special occasion.

Accepting individual large gifts, money or possessions left in a will is always unacceptable. If you are aware that a person intends to formally leave money to you, always report this to your manager. There are legal ways in which a person can donate to an organisation that will be used to enhance services to other clients.

Security in the home

Always take care when leaving a person's home to ensure that you have left them safe and that you close doors adequately. Remember that your own safety should also be considered, particularly if working alone on dark mornings or evenings. Your employing organisation should always have a record of the visits that you will be undertaking each day. Your line manager should always have an idea of when you can be expected to return or phone in.

If you hold keys to a client's home, these should ideally be signed out and signed back in after your working day. A locked key safe, with the keys identifiable by number or letter rather than the person's name will ensure greater security. This may not always be practical and you must therefore safeguard keys as if they were to your own home, and never write the client's name or address on the key label.

Conclusion

The legislation framework within which you will work imposes particular duties on managers and employing organisations. It is important that you are also aware of the implications and the way in which you can safeguard yourself and your client when carrying out duties. The legislation exists to protect everyone involved in providing and receiving care. Although it may be quicker to ignore some rules and policies the outcome may be tragic; most legislation exists because it has been proved there is a need for it.

Points to remember

1. Being aware of relevant legislation that safeguards individual rights is an impor-

tant part of providing care to people living in their own homes.

2. Each of us possesses personal rights to independence, to make decisions, to take risks and not to be discriminated against.

3. You should be aware of the broad areas of your work covered by legislation.

4. By promoting safe working environments and practices the health and safety of the clients receiving care and the people providing care can be protected.

5. It is unlawful to discriminate against anyone because of their gender or race.

6. Everyone has a right to know what personal information and data is recorded and kept about them in any form.

7. You may be at risk if exposed to harmful or hazardous substances. Always follow procedures and wear protective clothing where appropriate.

8. Where there is the risk of injury, every effort should be taken to redesign or avoid the task so that the risk of injury is reduced or removed.

9. Always resist getting involved with a person's finances unless you have been designated to undertake this duty by your employing authority.

10. The personal safety of your client and yourself is paramount at all times.

NVQ Levels 2 & 3 Core Units
O Promote equality for all individuals.
Z1 Contribute to the protection of individuals from abuse.
U4 Contribute to the health, safety and security or individuals and their environment.
U5 Obtain, store and transmit information relating to the delivery of a care service.
Level 2 Core Unit
W2 Contribute to the ongoing support of clients and others significant to them.
Level 3 Core Unit
Y2 Enable clients to make use of available services and information.
Level 2 Domiciliary Support
Y1 Enable clients to manage their domestic and personal resources.
U1 Contribute to the maintenance and management of domestic and personal resources.

CHAPTER 3

Promoting equality and anti-discriminatory practice

Judith Hodgkinson

• What is discrimination? • How does discrimination affect a care assistant's work? • Working with people from different cultural backgrounds • Issues for care assistants from Black and ethnic minorities • Promoting equality in face to face work • A framework for anti-discriminatory practice

One of the criteria for measuring the quality of our work is our willingness to deliver services tailor-made for each individual according to their needs and wishes – and for this we need discrimination. To be discriminating is to be able to perceive difference, which is no bad thing for a care worker.

In developing anti-discriminatory practice we are addressing the problem that because of their difference, some people are discriminated *against*. They are, in other words, treated as less than equal. Sometimes this is very obvious, but often it is happening in subtle ways. Sometimes we don't see it at all, and then when we look from a different angle we can see it very clearly.

If you are already employed as a care assistant in the community then you probably had to convince your interviewers that you believe all people should be treated equally. Unfortunately, in the translation from word to deed, such

beliefs can revert to "being nice to people if they're OK". So, if we don't critically examine what we're doing, it's all too easy to discriminate against all sorts of people who don't fit into our definition of "OK" (which very often means "like me/us").

We need to look carefully at how we behave with the people we work with. Developing anti-discriminatory practice has something to tell us about the way we work with *all* our clients, and it has something to offer us as workers because as we all know, discrimination doesn't just flow in one direction.

Discrimination in our work

Think up at least 12 reasons why people, whether clients or workers, experience adverse discrimination. Write them down before you move on. If you get stuck, don't give up. Think of your colleagues, clients and yourself: what are the sorts of things which create, or would create, inequalities in the way you treat each other and are treated by the organisation.

This was my list, also rapidly drawn up and incomplete:

- Disability
- Age
- Sexual orientation
- Class
- Race
- Religion
- Politics
- Accent
- Dress
- Personal habits/lifestyle
- Reputation (eg "difficult")
- Financial status
- Manner
- Having an infectious disease
- Making complaints

Try putting some of the reasons mentioned above into the first gap in the sentence below. Think about what your prejudices are as you do so, then you can fill in the second gap with the consequences of this prejudice:

"I understand you are... so I assume you are probably less..."

You might for example have thought of "I understand you are *young* so I assume you are probably less *reliable*" or "I understand you are *old* so I assume you are probably less *able to make your own decisions/aware of your rights/in need of privacy/flexible/likely to complain about me...*".

It is of real value to care assistants to take advantage of training courses on equal opportunities, or to read and study these issues for themselves. Courses can be found which explore key areas such as disability, equality, ageism and racism. If you have the opportunity to work towards an NVQ, anti-discriminatory practice will be seen as an essential part of your performance in every area. This chapter is an introduction to the issue.

Disability and older age

Thinking about disability or age as a cause of discrimination might seem like a contradiction when perhaps most of our clients will be older people and/or people with disabilities. After all, they are the reason the organisation exists: they are in the majority. This fact does not however overturn by itself the negative prejudices and assumptions about disability and age which are so dominant in our society.

Now and again the clients and carers we work with experience these negative images of themselves, and feel they aren't worth much. They can then disrespect you for wanting to work with them, or envy you for having a job, or be so grateful for any assistance that you can take advantage of them, bend the rules and rely on their compliance.

This is why it is so important that the organisation has clear guidelines for conduct for both you and your clients. Written guidelines minimise those areas which are open to discretion and interpretation, and are a protection for everyone if properly applied.

Race

Domiciliary care services often have difficulty attracting clients from black and ethnic minorities, for what may be a variety of reasons. Being aware of some of these reasons is useful when you come to work directly with black clients or those from minority cultures within society.

Faced with ageing, illness or disability, black people can experience particularly acute isolation, exacerbated by racism and hostility from some elements in the population. Sometimes people may not seek help because they are too depressed or (due to past experience) too wary of being poorly treated or misunderstood. Many older people from black and ethnic minorities are deeply disappointed because their dreams, perhaps of returning home, have not been realised.

In some cultures the stigma attached to disability, and mental illness particularly, mean that people strongly resist exposing their need for support. Often families hold a strong belief that they should be able to manage without any additional help, even from community services.

Sometimes the problem is one of language. People don't hear about services because they aren't informed through appropriate channels. Or even when they try services, what they receive will be less satisfactory if they can't get the guidelines translated or make their wishes properly understood, either at assessment or to you, the care worker.

Equal opportunities at work

The agency you work for should actively recruit workers to reflect the ethnic mix of the population it serves, so that the demand for appropriate languages can be met. People with dementia for example can revert to using their first language exclusively and will benefit from a worker who understands them. Such efforts though, can only ever be partially effective within the necessary frameworks of limited financial resources, and employment policies which seek to offer everyone a fair and equal chance of employment – regardless of race, dress code and so on.

So while managers can always try to match workers and clients they think will have something in common – be it religion, experience, sexual preferences or that Glasgow accent – the equal opportunities approach must be upheld. This means that just as you, the worker, must be prepared to work with anyone who accepts and abides by the conditions of the service, so clients need to accept

workers in the same light: people working to the same job description and standards.

You could therefore find yourself working with someone from a religious or ethnic background historically antagonistic to your own. In your professional role it is essential that you strive to lay these issues aside, respect the equal value of each human being and recognise our shared human needs.

HIV positive

If a client or colleague is known or suspected to be HIV positive they can be discriminated against, frequently because of the ignorance and fear of those responsible about how the virus is transmitted. The fear and ignorance can be very successfully dispelled through education and clear policies on safe practices (hygiene and infection control) In this instance, it is important to assume that everyone is HIV positive and therefore each person will be treated in the same way. We should have the same attitudes, infection control policy and provide the same care – particularly when we do not know a person's HIV status.

Lifestyles

In the list we made before of reasons why people can be discriminated against, you will see that some can stem from the way people choose to live, as well as from the things they can't change. These types of things have included, in my experience, how clean or otherwise their living accommodation is, how they spend their money, the type of relationship they have with the person they care for or are cared for by, or the hours they keep.

It is clear that while a care assistant will inevitably notice such things and may need occasionally to give vent to their feelings about them to a supervisor, such feelings should not affect their work or their behaviour towards clients and carers in any way.

Nor should these personal details find their way into any other conversations with either friends or colleagues. It is hard enough for people who need services to accept assistance and to have someone in their home with access to the personal details of their daily lives. One of your most serious responsibilities as a care assistant is not to betray the trust that has been placed in you but to respect the confidential nature of all these details.

Likewise any discussion about your colleagues and managers with clients which divulges information they don't need to know, or encourages gossip, can be extremely harmful and should be firmly avoided. Your employer should give you the opportunity to discuss the grey areas of confidentiality at staff meetings to strengthen you in this aspect of anti-discriminatory practice.

Different backgrounds

When you work with people from backgrounds different to your own, it is worth taking the trouble to find out about the things which are likely to be important to them. Your library might have useful information, or your local Voluntary Action Council may, like mine, have published profiles of the area which go some way to increasing one's understanding. Local community organisations can be approached directly for information – your local authority should have lists of these.

But remember that you can still assume nothing about the individual you are working with unless you have checked it out with them first. Beware too of assuming that people are traditional, or indeed that they wish to convey their traditional values to you. It is likely that most of your clients will be concerned with the here and now realities of life, and happier to discuss these with newcomers. Do not forget that as residents of the same region there will be issues which concern you both. Perhaps too many of us have come to expect that giving support to a person entitles us to know about their past, to be intimate, to counsel, to intervene. A spell working for an adult individual with physical disabilities, solely under their direction and in their own home should perhaps be compulsory retraining for domiciliary care workers in this respect, especially those of us used to working in residential settings. (See also chapter 4, Multicultural health needs).

Challenging racism

We live in a society where there is much movement and change in our perceptions, and within which it is possible to say that harmony and disharmony co-exist – between men and women, young and old, rich and poor, and between different racial groups. Racism is common. Frequently black workers will deny personal experience of racism and take particular pride in the evidence of their clients' appreciation.

However some black care assistants will eventually, if they feel secure, reveal that early encounters with some clients have indeed been frosty and unpleasant. If you suspect that a client has rejected you on racial grounds you should ask your manager to investigate. Most organisations will refuse to accept discrimination from clients on these grounds, and service should be withdrawn. Exceptions to this would be where a service user has a mental impairment such as dementia. The risk of rejection can be minimised in this and all situations, if a new worker is introduced in person to the client by someone well known and trusted, for example an existing worker.

You may suspect that you are being discriminated against in fairly subtle ways by your manager, and this can be just as hard to deal with. In some teams it always seems to be the black workers who are given the unpopular clients. White workers may, for a range of reasons, be able to be assertive about what they aren't prepared to do and the manager may find it easier to allow this situation to continue rather than challenge it. Similarly you may feel that you are being offered less work if your manager tries to avoid problems by not sending you to a client he or she suspects could be racist.

Your manager may not even be conscious of these practices, but they need to be challenged. Try to win support in your team and management for bringing these issues into the open. Careful monitoring of recruitment and work allocation will be necessary. Your local authority may have a race equality unit which can get involved, or you can use your trades union.

Most service providers are now dependent on contracts and service agreements with their local authorities for at least part of their income and the local authority will be interested if it appears that an organisation with which it has a contract is not following an equal opportunities policy in any aspect of service provision or staff management.

Promoting equality

In order to effectively discriminate against others, you need to have power in relation to them. Thus in order to promote equality you will need to be aware of where the power lies in the context of your work.

If you are delivering a service on behalf of a local authority or a charity then the service is likely to be free or subsidised.

People may now receive services paid for by the local authority but provided by a private, profit-making agency. Historically the provision of free health and social services has put clients into a fairly vulnerable position, with service providers making the key decisions – and monopolising provision, of course, so that there has been little real choice.

As a care assistant, you can be placed in a very powerful position if your client feels:
• that they are lucky to have a service,
• if they feel very dependent on it,
• if there is no alternative, or they know of no alternative,
• if they feel that to complain would incur the wrath and resentment of staff which would go unchecked,
• if they have not been made aware of their rights as consumers or of the standards they can expect,
• if they do not have the ability to exercise their rights and lack an advocate who can act on their behalf.

Changing the balance of power can be achieved to a large extent by putting each of these things right and more. How far any of this has been achieved in your work setting is something it would be useful for you to consider.

For workers paid directly by clients, or employed by an agency paid directly by the client, the power in the relationship is more clear cut, although as an employer the client will need stamina, mental capacity and experience – or an advocate who can act on their behalf. The power to hire and fire can be the surest way for some people who need personal assistance of making their wishes count. A care assistant might not wave the talcum powder about quite so freely, because "It's what we do", in spite of the protestations of the carer at her elbow who insists "But Mother's always hated the stuff" – if Mother or the carer could put her out of a job the next day.

Experience has shown that direct employment of workers is too risky, time consuming and fraught a method of service provision for all but a minority of people needing services. As a care assistant it is also important to be aware that people with disabilities are no more benign as direct employers than the rest of the population and that there are significant safeguards and advantages for workers in being part of an organisation.

Those people with disabilities involved with agencies offering services for independent living should, however, have the opportunity to co-manage their own care packages and from this experience some will wish to move on to being a direct employer.

For most however a managing organisation has huge advantages such as continuity, relief cover, recruitment and administration, health and safety policy, insurance, training, staff supervision and support and a mediator when there are difficulties.

There is evidence then that without sufficient safeguards and accountability, clients can experience adverse discrimination and lack power as service consumers.

Who has the power?

The way a care assistant behaves in face to face work with a client really counts, and will probably reflect their perception of the service user's power or lack of it. But by becoming more aware of the way you are with a client you can get more than half way towards changing it. Often "training" will not achieve this change in you because it tries to teach you "correct" skills without enabling you to look at and critically examine your own beliefs and practice first.

The following are some cartoons in words, depicting some of the different ways a care assistant can be. See if you can work out where the care assistant is holding power and how. Can you recognise anyone you know here?

The brisk parental approach: "Can we get on with it?"

The easily offended approach: "You don't need to tell me what to do if he has a fit – I'm an experienced carer."

The non-assertive, out of my depth, half-there approach: "I'm hanging about, not saying much. I don't know what to do but I don't like to ask. I'd rather be somewhere else anyway." or: "If I keep quiet and don't look you in the eye we can avoid your grief and pain."

The exploitative: "I'll put the TV on shall I? Can't miss Home and Away, it's got to an exciting bit." or "I've got a lot of problems too and if I tell you about them you'll help me out by not telling anyone that I'm always late."

The angel of mercy/friend for life approach: "I'll give you my phone number, in case you need someone to talk to, but don't tell the office." or "I'm a caring person, my clients love me. I go to see one of them in hospital and I cry to her 'Don't talk about dying, I couldn't bear to lose you'."

The downright insulting: "Am I glad to see you. These four hours with your mother are so boring."

The expert: "This is how I'm going to lift you. I know what feels good for you because I've been trained."

The frantically busy and self important approach: "Hello, I'll just leave my shopping here by the door. When I've had my sandwiches we could have a quick game of cards if you like but can I leave ten minutes early because the buses are all to pot and I've got to pick the kids up. What a day, you've no idea. Oh, nearly forgot, can I make a quick phone call."

Manipulation

These examples show how workers can be manipulative. It is interesting that those workers who are too caring and those who lack assertiveness can disempower a service user as effectively as those whose bid for control is more direct. The client finds herself looking after the shy worker or can't be at ease with her; a worker who needs constant direction and reassurance is not adequately meeting needs but can make a client feel guilty about criticising or make it almost impossible for such things to be said. The angel of mercy who cares too much achieves an even greater stranglehold on the client because if they do criticise or try to make changes it becomes a rejection of love. The client's rights can become very blurred; this one even has to feel guilty about dying!

You do not have to be highly experienced or know about every type of problem to be confident as a care assistant. Your clients will be impressed by your respect for them and for how they want things done; by being there for them, rather than preoccupied with other things; perhaps by the calm your arrival can bring to a fraught situation.

Empowerment

If you can be assertive and open with clients, you are in effect setting free those who would otherwise find it difficult to say what they need, request changes in the way things are done without apologising, point out when standards aren't being met without fearing that the relationship will collapse, and of course, have first class personal assistance without the added burden of your loving care.

What does being open and assertive sound like?

"Would you like to tell me, when you're ready, the things you think I need to know."

"Tell me how you like this to be done."

"I'm finding the cigarette smoke a bit difficult now. Could I step out onto the balcony for a minute or shall I open a window?"

"We didn't make the apricot whip today because your mother wanted to spend longer on the foot bath. Also I didn't finish the washing up as she wasn't happy. We had a look at the photos again instead. I felt it was the best decision for today but I wanted to ask you how you felt about it."

"I think I might have damaged the television. I'm really sorry if that's the case. This is what happened..."

Framework for practice

• Care assistants and clients should be working to an equal opportunities policy which is actively monitored and pursued.

• Both workers and clients should know their rights and what is expected of them. These rights need to be written and made available to people when they start their involvement with the organisation and there should be the opportunity to discuss them with a manager. They should be translated where necessary.

• The organisation should be internally and externally monitored so that it is accountable to consumers, local authorities and funders where applicable.

Staff

• require a written grievance procedure

• should have written guidelines about what they can expect from users and how to conduct themselves when working in people's homes

• should have the chance to meet and make recommendations/give feedback on

the policy and development of the organisation
• should have training and support to develop anti-discriminatory practice.

Clients

• should have a clear complaints procedure and should be told at the initial assessment of the organisation's commitment to taking complaints seriously
• should have guidelines which show what tasks workers can be expected to do and what the conditions of service are, in terms for example of treatment of workers
• should have the opportunity to review the service they receive, and their own role as clients, according to an agreed written format, together with a service manager or a third party at regular intervals. The review should address the workings of the equal opportunities policy as well as all other aspects of the service. Agreements made at these reviews should be made available in writing to clients.
• should have representation within the organisation and be consulted on key issues. Their participation in the management of the organisation should be encouraged as far as possible through appropriate training, including equal opportunities training, and through practical support. It should be made possible for clients to meet as a group from time to time to make this representation effective.

Points to remember

1. Promoting equality is about recognising and accepting differences, not ignoring them.
2. Even when people seem to invite you to patronise them, don't do it.

3. Disclosing confidential information about clients or colleagues, especially to each other, destroys any attempt to construct equality in this type of relationship. Do not abuse your position.
4. Confront your own ignorance and complacency about other lifestyles and cultures; find out all you can. But don't assume anything about an individual unless you have checked it with them first.
5. Having written standards of practice and procedure in your organisation will give both workers and clients a good measure of protection against prejudice and discrimination. You could search out those used by other organisations to encourage your employers to improve yours.
6. Be assertive and clear with clients and carers as a mark of your respect for them. This will set them free to be the same with you.
7. Equality isn't a side issue. Put the promotion of equality at the centre of your work as a care assistant, and you'll see the difference!

NVQ Level 2 & 3 Core Units
O Promote equality for all individuals.
Z1 Contribute to the protection of individuals from abuse.
U4 Contribute to the health, safety and security of individuals and their environment.
U5 Obtain, transmit and store information relating to the delivery of a care service.

Level 2 Core Unit
W2 Contribute to the ongoing support of clients and others significant to them.

Level 3 Core Units
Z4 Promote communication with clients where there are comunication difficultiies.
Y2 Enable clients to make use of available services and information.

Level 2 Domiciliary Support
W8 Enable clients to maintain contacts in potentially isolating situations.

CHAPTER 4

Multicultural care needs

Mansour Jumaa

- *Individually focused care that takes account of different cultural needs*
- *Food and diet* • *Practical care* • *Family planning* • *Ethnicity and illness*
- *Spiritual care* • *Dying and death*

People from Black and minority ethnic groups need the same respect, friendly and individually focused care as any other client. They may also have special care needs which stem from their cultural or religious background. Knowledge of these areas will help you give better, more individual care – provided that you remember that everyone is different, and it would be as wrong to lump together all Muslims (for example) as the same, as to ignore their special needs altogether.

You should try to find out as much as possible about an individual's habits and preferences from them, their family and/or friends, and you may well need help from them or a representative of their community if there are language or communication problems.

I hope this chapter will raise your awareness of differences between your own beliefs, practices and expectations, and those of your clients from different cultural backgrounds. It focuses on the following areas:
- Food and diets
- Family planning
- Practical care
- Ethnicity and illness
- Spiritual care
- Dying and death

Food and diet

Food and diet needs of people from other cultures are usually but not always dictated by their religious beliefs and practices. If you are involved in preparing meals or helping a person to eat pre-cooked foods, it is essential that you are aware of the following:

Muslim people are not allowed to eat pork. All meat must be slaughtered according to the Halal ritual. This ritual ensures that the blood of the meat is drained. Devout Muslims may want to fast (no intake of food or drink between sunrise and sunset) during the month of Ramadan. Those who are sick are not compelled to fast. Muslims are also forbidden to eat shellfish and eels, but may eat fish that have fins and scales.

Jewish clients also are not allowed to eat any pig products. They may eat only animals that have been ritually slaughtered in the Jewish tradition (Kosher). Meat and milk dishes are never allowed to be mixed within the same meal. In fact Jews will be offended if offered pig meat in any form.

Like the **Rastafarians**, many **Buddhist** clients are vegetarians. Alcohol is strictly prohibited for Rastafarians, and some follow strict dietary restrictions similar to Jews. Many **Hindu** clients do not eat meat and are forbidden to kill any animal, especially the cow. Hindus who are vegetarians cannot eat off a plate on which meat has previously being served.

Most **Sikh** women are vegetarians, and may also exclude egg and fish from their diet. Those (very few) who eat meat will not eat beef. So it is especially important to explain to a client what a particular dish – eg "hotpot" – contains.

Ensuring that clients from different cultural backgrounds have access to appropriate diets will help to maintain a sense of cultural identity which is vital to their self-esteem.

Practical care

Knowledge will enable you to be sensitive to specific health beliefs and practices. How would you, for example, interpret the bland refusal of an **Orthodox Jew** to shake hands with you? You are a care worker and female. The explanation may be that Orthodox Jews may not have any physical contact with women in case they are currently menstruating. Even within marriage, a husband and wife may not be able to pass an object directly from one to another without first putting it down.

Hindu, Sikh, and **Muslim** women are likely to have a strong preference to be seen or treated by a female health care worker. Other individuals, especially elderly people, may also not allow someone of the opposite sex to see them undressed.

Afro Caribbean people have specific skin and hair care requirements, requiring hair gels and oils in order to prevent their hair becoming matted and their skin dry and sore. Many **Asian** women always cover their hair and their legs. **Sikh** men always wear turbans and these are not removed.

Washing and bathing

We all know that hygiene and cleanliness are essential in maintaining health. Yet experience suggests that many health care workers always want to impose their own principles of hygiene and cleanliness. It is crucial for effective care to accept that people from different cultural backgrounds also have different but equally valid, and sometimes better, principles of hygiene.

For example, many **Asian** clients do not like to bathe because they see this as sitting in dirty water; they prefer to rinse themselves with clean water.

For religious, personal, and or moral reasons, hygiene may be neglected or actively encouraged; rituals of washing and purification may be carried out on a regular basis, as in the case of devout **Muslims**; and bathing arrangements may be private or communal. Unless you have evidence to show how these practices could be harmful, you should sensitively support them.

Family planning

In this section we look at the family planning and childbirth practices of clients from multicultural and multiracial backgrounds. Like all other areas, these issues are very sensitive. Be cautious and treat your clients with respect and dignity. In the UK, and indeed in the western world, the debate on abortion and family planning centres around the right of the woman to control her own body and fertility. But in some cultures and communities, a man is entirely responsible for his wife and children, as well as decisions on family planning. Should you have enough evidence that a woman's health may be put in danger by another pregnancy, you may need to discuss this with her husband. A male health care worker is the most suitable person to manage this discussion wherever possible. If the family is devout in its practice of rituals and health beliefs, mixed sex discussions on contraception should be discouraged. You are unlikely to achieve anything if your clients feel embarrassed and uncomfortable.

Muslims, Jews, Rastafarians and Roman Catholics regard artificial contraception methods as contrary to the teachings of their religion. Rastafarians, like Jews, may hold strongly to the Old Testament teaching: "Be fruitful, and multiply, and replenish the earth" (Genesis 1:28).

There are also political issues of which you need to be aware. You need to ask yourself, for example, what is behind Third World family planning programmes? Is it an attempt to increase the control that these women will have over their own lives, and to liberate them from an endless cycle of pregnancy and childbirth? Or is it really an attempt to force birth control on certain targeted sections of the population? How, for example, would you react to a Rastafarian family in the community who are reluctant to limit their families? Their argument is that family planning is an example of white oppression of black people.

Ethnicity and illness

There are specific illness conditions which affect people in the UK who are members of Black and ethnic minority groups. The most common conditions are listed below; more information is given in the publications listed at the end of this chapter.

Ethnic origin/common disease
Asian
Rickets and osteomalacia
European Jewish
Tay-Sachs disease
Mediterranean, North Africa and Asian
Thalassaemia
Northern and Central Europe
Cystic fibrosis
African and Afro-Caribbean
Sickle cell disease

Spiritual care

Do not assume that all spiritual care has to be dictated by religion. Strong personal beliefs that the individual finds comforting may form the basis of their spiritual wellbeing. Nevertheless, the spiritual care needed by most clients from different racial backgrounds is dictated by their religious beliefs.

Worship and prayer
Worship and prayer play a vital part in the life of religious people of all faiths. Each person will have their own specific prayer and worship needs. Devout **Muslims**, for example, will want to pray undisturbed five times a day at special prayer times from early morning to late evening.

All staff must be aware of a person's religious requirements, and must accept that this aspect of their life is very important to their wellbeing.

Some **Sikhs** chose to "take Amrit" (a kind of confirmation) and are therefore bound to observe special rules, for example the wearing of the "Five Ks": Kesh – uncut hair; Kangha – the wooden comb; Kara – iron wrist band; Kirpan – a short sword; and Kach – short trousers/breeches. These symbols should not be disturbed nor laughed at.

Pain

Pain may be private (not visible to others) or public. Pain can also serve many purposes: social, physiological, psychological and spiritual. The spiritual aspect of pain differs among different cultural and racial groups. This means that they may respond to pain in ways we don't expect. We may, for example, assume that painkilling drugs are working, when in fact the person is uncomplaining because they feel they should have to suffer.

Dying and death

People from different racial backgrounds have religious practices which must be followed for the care of the dying and the preparation of the dead.

A dying **Muslim** client may wish to sit or lie facing towards Mecca. He or she will also appreciate recitation of Prayers from the Holy Koran by another Muslim. Dying **Jews** may appreciate hearing special psalms, such as Psalm 23, and the special prayer (the Sherma). A dying **Sikh** may receive comfort from reciting hymns from Guru Grant Sahab, the Sikh Holy Book. Similarly, hymns and readings from Bhagavad Gita, one of the Hindu Holybooks, may be a source of comfort to a devout **Hindu** who is dying. Some people may request to lie on the floor – a symbolic gesture of closeness to Mother Earth.

After death

If the client dies, certain practices must be carried out, some of which are listed below. Through discussion with relatives staff should know how to contact a local religious leader if this is desired.

Religious practices at death

ISLAM

No part of the body must be cut out, harmed or donated to anyone else. Devout Muslims will not agree to organ transplants. Non-Muslims must NOT touch the body. Always wear disposable gloves. Do not wash the body, nor cut hair or nails. Seek more details from the qualified registered practitioner. Funeral is preferred within 24 hours. Always buried, never cremated, with the head facing Mecca.

HINDUISM

If permission was previously sought, no religious objections to organ transplantation. Non-Hindus must NOT touch the body. Do not remove jewellery, sacred threads and other religious objects. Wrap in a plain sheet without religious emblem. Relatives will wash the body. Adult Hindus are cremated. Infants and children may be buried. Funeral must take place as soon as possible.

JUDAISM

No objection in principle to organ transplant, provided no organ is removed until death is definitely established. Body to be handled as little as possible by others. Burial, preferably within 24 hours of death; only delayed for the Sabbath. Orthodox Jews are always buried.

BUDDHISM

No objection to blood transfusion or organ transplant. Ritualistic requirements almost nil. Very important that you inform a Buddhist minister or monk of the same school of Buddhism as the deceased, as soon as possible. The body should be disposed of in three to seven days. Most prefer cremation.

SIKHISM

No objections to organ transplant. Non-Sikhs are allowed to tend the body, and perform the normal last offices, if the family wishes. However, in Sikh tradition the family is responsible for all ceremonies and death rites, so if they are available, consult them. Do NOT trim hair or beard. Sikhs are always cremated, except stillbirths and new-born babies who may be buried. Cremation should take place within 24 hours.

Respect for individuals

As always, remember that every client is an individual: delivering stereotyped care because they are from a certain culture would be as bad as ignoring their cultural needs altogether. One of the most important things to remember is that each client will follow their religion to different degrees. Each client will still have their own personal needs, and will have their own way of living their faith.

Your role in providing care is the same as for any other client, with a special regard for any specific needs. You must not judge patients because of their beliefs or customs, and must always respect those beliefs and traditions.

You also need to understand that elderly people from the Black and ethnic minority groups expect some respect from the younger generations. Bear this in mind and you will be able to form an effective working relationship with them.

Points to remember

1. People from different cultural backgrounds may have special care needs, **but** don't assume that an individual will follow all the traditional customs and practices of their ethnic or cultural community.
2. Respect and don't discourage traditional beliefs and practices unless they have been proved to be harmful.
3. Be aware of how your own cultural values may prejudice you.
4. Always be sensitive and find out the prevalent attitudes within the community towards family planning.
5. A relationship of mutual confidence built up over time between a woman and a particular health care worker will be more acceptable.
6. Try to work with individuals to fulfill their spiritual needs in a positive way.
7. When caring for a dying person, ensure that you are familiar with special preparation, and cultural ceremonies, relevant to their or their family's wishes.
8. Do not be frightened to raise the awareness of other staff who may not know what the individual has requested.

Resources

Mares P, Henley A, Baxter C (1984) *Healthcare in a Multiracial Britain*. Health Education Council/National Extension College, London.
Squires AJ (Ed) (1991) *Multicultural Health Care and Rehabilitation of Older People*. Age Concern/Edward Arnold.
Pami Bal *Health Needs of a Multi-Racial Population* £4.99 from Liverpool Helath Authority Community and Priority Services Unit, Sefton General Hospital, Smithdown Road, Liverpool L15 2HE.
Collins, D. Tank, M. Basith, A. (1993) *Concise Guide to Customs of Minority Ethnic Religions*. Arena Aldershot.

NVQ Levels 2 & 3 Core Units
O Promote equality for all individuals.
U4 Contribute to the health, safety and security of individuals and their environment.
U5 Obtain, transmit and store information relating to the delivery of a care service.
Level 2 Core Unit
W2 Contribute to the ongoing support of clients and others significant to them.
Level 3 Core Units
Z4 Promote communication with clients where there are communication difficulties.
Y2 Enable clients to make use of available services and information.
Level 2 Direct Care
Z10 Enable clients to eat and drink.
Z11 Enable clients to access and use toilet facilities.
Level 2 Domiciliary Support
W8 Enable clients to maintain contacts in potentially isolating situations.

CHAPTER 5

Talking and listening

Jane Maxim and Karen Bryan

• How to convey information clearly and be a good listener
• Using your eyes as well as your ears • Different ways of speaking • Language barriers • How being ill or disabled affects communication • Stroke and language disorders • Elderly people • Dementia • Mental illness • Learning disability • Talking to children • How to help people with hearing problems

What is communication? What can make communication difficult? What can be done to make communication easier?

It is often said that someone is a good communicator when they can talk well and interest their listener. But there are two sides to good communication: being able to make the meaning clear *and* being able to listen and understand what is being said.

For most people, good communication is an important part of their daily life. For people who are ill or disabled, perhaps restricted to bed, who may be very anxious about their health and wellbeing, communication is particularly important.

As well as conveying their needs and asking questions, many people will welcome the opportunity to talk about their worries. They will also want to hear and to talk about what is happening outside their own home environment.

Look and listen

Communication is the process of conveying information between two or more people. Communication involves talking, listening, writing and reading, facial expression, gesture and body language. Thoughts are put into words and sentences to convey meaning. Speech is produced by co-ordinated muscle movements of the larynx, tongue and face. But part of the message is conveyed by other means:

• hand and body movements to produce gestures such as shrugging the shoulders
• changes in voice and pitch, for example we describe someone as "sounding" angry
• the use of facial expression such as a smile or frown.

The listener needs to listen to the actual words spoken **and** attend to the other information that the speaker is conveying, in order to fully appreciate the meaning. So listening involves using your eyes as well as your ears.

Different ways of speaking

People vary tremendously in the way they speak. Men sound different from women and people have a wide range of different accents (the way we speak) and dialects (what words we use and the way we use them). In addition, we all vary the way we speak depending on who we are speaking to and the circumstances of the conversation. Most of the time we do this without even being aware of it.

To take an example, the way in which we speak to a colleague at work is very different to the way in which we speak to a baby or young child. With a colleague we have a shared knowledge of the job to be done and use the appropriate vocabulary for that situation. We are speaking to someone whom we assume will understand what we are saying without any need for us to change the way we speak. However, if we were explaining part of the job to somebody who was not familiar with it, then the type and amount of information we give would vary.

It is important that when you talk to clients, you give them the right amount of information: too little and they will not understand you, too much and they will feel that you are treating them as if they are stupid.

• Be sensitive to the different ways people speak.

• Be aware of how you are speaking yourself.

• Don't jump to hasty assumptions about people just because of the way they sound.

It is also important not to assume that people who are ill or in some way disabled are automatically incapable of normal understanding and speaking. The people you will encounter in your work may have differing styles of speech. Some people have very quiet voices, others very loud ones, someone may be used to speaking in short, abrupt phrases while other people may talk at great length with lots of detail.

• Communication difficulty leads to immense frustration.

• It often gains the person the label of being "difficult"

• Communication difficulty can also affect relationships with other people, including family and friends, and can lead to social isolation.

Language barriers

Most people have experienced difficulty in communicating while on holiday in another country. A simple task such as buying a railway ticket can become almost impossible when two people do not speak, understand, read or write the same language. There are many people in Britain who live within communities where little or in some cases no English is spoken. In order to make communication easier:

• watch the person's facial expression and gestures as these may convey some of the meaning

• try to anticipate their needs, for example by looking around them to see if anything is wrong

• speak to the person in a normal voice at a normal speed, but use short sentences and attempt to convey only the important points

• use gestures as you speak, for example "Do you want a drink?" can be accompanied by a mime of drinking

• try to find out about the person from their family or friends, who may be able to help by writing down some key words for you with a translation, and can tell you a little about the person, the way they are feeling and any particular dislikes they may have

• if the person has no family or carer who

can help, try to find a member of staff or a neighbour or friend who can speak the same language. Most health and local authority departments have advocacy and interpreting services and a list of staff who speak other languages.

How illness affects us

Imagine how you might feel if you were ill or disabled and alone at home: very unsure about what is happening, worrying about what will happen next, feeling ill, uncomfortable, or in pain. All these factors are bound to affect the way a person communicates with others.

Some people may react by being over-cheerful and trying to convince everyone else that they are not at all worried; others may become very quiet and withdrawn; others may be abstracted and so appear not to really know what is happening; others may be very forceful and angry, perhaps about trivial things. Therefore it is important to think about why a person may speak to you in a way that you don't expect.

All this means that you must try to:

• approach clients carefully in a sensitive manner

• react calmly to the client

• be sympathetic to their situation

• have some understanding of why they may react oddly.

As well as all of the factors mentioned above, many clients may have specific difficulties in communicating. All the problems described in the following sections of this chapter will affect clients' ability to communicate normally. It is important to consider the impact on a person of not being able to communicate normally. It will lead to:

• difficulty in expressing immediate wants, for example to go to the toilet

> **Coping with anger:**
> • accept that the person is expressing strong feelings and do not try to contradict or belittle these feelings
> • give the person a chance to discuss how they are feeling and what is really upsetting them so that you can try to understand the situation
> • speak calmly and gently and offer reassurance once the outburst is over

• difficulty in expressing feelings such as sadness, anger

• difficulty in expressing needs, for example to see a particular member of their family.

Anxiety and embarrassment

Anxiety or worry can obviously cause a person to react in an unexpected way. Embarrassment can also lead to this. A previously independent person may be very embarrassed by needing help with, for example, toileting.

It is important that although *you* have become used to nursing and care routines, you do not forget that these can be strange or even seem degrading to some people. It is therefore important to explain what is being done and why, and to understand the reasons why someone might be uncooperative or even get angry with you.

Anger and abuse

A client who is angry may even show this by shouting at you, possibly by verbal abuse such as swearing and, especially if they have difficulty in talking, by trying to push you away or even throwing something towards you.

Remember to remain calm and try to understand what is happening. Often the person has been gradually becoming more frustrated, perhaps by their restricted mobility, or maybe they are really upset because their family have not visited. Or perhaps they have just been told bad news about their medical condition. (See also chapter 20 on inappropriate and antisocial behaviour.)

Stroke

Clients who have had a stroke (cerebrovascular accident), often have difficulties in communicating which can persist for years afterwards. *Dysphasia* and *dysarthria* are the most common problems.

> **Dysphasia is a language disorder which may affect understanding, speaking, reading and writing.**
>
> **Dysarthria is a speech disorder caused by poor muscle movement or poor muscle coordination.**

Dysphasia

Stroke can damage certain areas of the brain which cause an adult to have an acquired language disorder, called dysphasia. In dysphasia the ability to understand and express meaning through words is disrupted. This may affect speech, reading and writing.

The exact effect of a stroke on speech and language will vary from one individual to another depending upon their injury, their previous education, work and experiences, their personality and their present communication needs relating to their environment. Dysphasic adults may have non-fluent speech: they have difficulty producing sentences or even words in severe cases. For example, they might say "doctor" where "I would like to see the doctor" might be expected, or "wu" for water.

Sometimes errors are made. These may involve changing sounds – "ted" for "bed" – or use of an incorrect word –"boy" for "girl". Other dysphasic people may have fluent speech but difficulty in finding the right words. For example:

"That's a, oh a, you know, tea, tea, drink it, no *cup*".

In other cases, although speech is fluent, it is not correctly structured so that little meaning is expressed.

A person's understanding of language can also be disrupted by dysphasia but not necessarily in the same way as their expressive speech. Reading and writing are usually affected in the same way as speech, but occasionally someone is able to write down what they cannot say.

Where possible a speech and language therapist can be asked to give details of a dysphasic person's speech and language abilities and to give specific advice on the most effective ways of achieving communication. Staff and carers can also observe a dysphasic person, noting the difficulties that they are having with communication, and what helps them.

The following general guidelines are helpful to remember when speaking to a dysphasic person:

• Slow down.

• Remove distractions (eg TV).

• Break any speech into stages. For example :

"It's getting cold, isn't it?"
"Are you cold?"
"Do you want a blanket?

• Try to understand the person. Asking questions which only need a yes/no answer may help to give you clues. For example "Is it sore?"

• Maintain contact with the person while they struggle to speak: look towards them, look interested and wait patiently.

• Give them time to speak.

• Commiserate with them if they become upset or frustrated.

• The person is not stupid; speaking loudly and slowly does not help. Use normal voice and expression.

• Ask the person's opinion.

• Use gesture – "Would you like a cup of coffee?" – point to the coffee pot while asking.

• Try to remember that speaking and understanding may be a great effort, so try to break up taking a case history etc. Do not expect a dysphasic person to talk for too long, and be alert to signs of fatigue.

Dysarthria

Problems with physically producing the sounds of speech can also occur after stroke and some other diseases such as Parkinson's disease, multiple sclerosis, and motor neurone disease.

This is called dysarthria and refers to a difficulty in speech production with no problems in understanding, reading or writing (unless another physical problem, such as arthritic fingers, affects these).

The main forms of dysarthria are:

Flaccid dysarthria: Here the muscles are weak and floppy. The person may have a very quiet voice making them sound difficult to hear, and their speech may sound unclear.

Spastic dysarthria: Here the muscles are very stiff, making movement difficult. Speech is therefore jerky with sudden changes in loudness.

Parkinsonian dysarthria: Here the muscles are stiff and unco-ordinated. This causes the person's speech to speed up, and the speech is often difficult to hear at the end of a sentence.

A person with dysarthria can understand language fully and has no problem in thinking what to say or in formulating a response in his head, but has a physical difficulty in speaking the words because the speech muscles are not working normally.

In some cases very little speech can be achieved, or the speech is unintelligible. However, it is often the case that people in everyday contact with a dysarthric speaker can "tune in" to their speech and understand them well. Some dysarthric people are able to use writing or a communication aid such as a pointing chart or an electronic device, to add to or replace their speech.

Elderly people

Elderly people essentially speak and understand in the same way as younger people. They may suffer from sensory losses such as reduced vision and hearing which can be corrected provided that glasses and hearing aids are worn. Teeth are also important for speech, so if dentures are used they should always be worn and should be regularly checked to ensure that they fit correctly.

> Is the elderly person
> • wearing cleaned glasses?
> • wearing a hearing aid in good working order?
> • wearing dentures that fit well?

However, research shows that elderly people hesitate and pause more when they speak. Older people say themselves that they sometimes find it difficult to remember a particular word, often a name. But everyone has this difficulty from time to time.

Elderly people may also be *slower* at

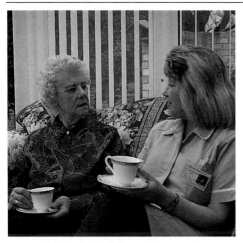

It is important to speak to older people exactly as you would speak to younger adults.

understanding what is said to them, although their actual ability to understand is not diminished. It is important therefore that you speak to older people as you would to younger adults. There is a tendency to speak to older people as if they are small children, which should be avoided.

Elderly people may of course suffer from specific diseases that can affect their ability to talk and understand in the same way as younger people.

Dementia

A minority of elderly people suffer from **dementia**, a gradual loss of brain cells resulting in progressive loss of memory, slowing of activity and difficulty with the tasks of everyday life (see chapter 13). Communication is also affected in dementia.

As the disease progresses, communication is affected by memory loss, and the ability to name people and objects is gradually reduced. The fluency of speech increases so that speech becomes rambling and fragmented. Here is an example from an eighty-two year old lady with a two-year history of dementia, describing a picture of a busy high street. She has been widowed for twenty years:

"Two ladies, baker, somebody leading a little baby. I had a little baby. I don't see much of my husband now. She turned around and looked at me. Supermarket".

Understanding becomes gradually more difficult and there may be problems with reading and writing.

In the later stages of dementia, speech reduces until the person only speaks occasional words. Some people also produce echo-speech, repeating what has been said to them. By this stage the person has severe problems with understanding and is probably only able to understand a few conversational points. Reading and writing become impossible.

It is obviously difficult to communicate verbally with a person suffering from advanced dementia. However, the early and middle stages can last for many years, and during this time effective communication can be achieved.

There are five basic points to consider in order to assist communication with someone who has a dementia:

1. Do not assume that any aspects of meaning which are not specified will be understood. For example, you may talk about the next meal and be very well aware that this must be breakfast because it is 7am and the elderly person is just getting up. But you must make this clear, by using the word "breakfast".

2. Be very direct – cut out any unnecessary details.

3. Keep the content direct. For example, the remark, "I imagine it's rather like flying" would be very difficult for a person with dementia to understand.

4. Do not assume that the person remembers; he or she is likely not to, even though what you refer to may be a daily event.

5. Try to give additional facial and gestural clues to assist understanding.

Mental illness

Mental functioning can be changed by physical diseases for which the cause is known, such as viruses or tumours that affect the brain. Other conditions which have unknown causes, such as depression, psychosis and neurosis, may affect the main areas of mental functioning, which are:

• **mood** which may be angry, happy, sad...

• **cognition** which includes the ability to think, remember, understand and learn

• **behaviour** which includes the way that we react, the tasks that we perform and the way we carry them out.

Changes in mental functioning can have a profound effect on communication. Much of what the person says may reflect the problems they are having in thinking and behaving normally. In other cases, such as severe depression, the person may rarely communicate or even become totally mute. Occasionally people suffering from mental illness can be verbally and physically abusive (see pages 39-40). It is important to try to find out about an individual with a mental illness, and the best way to approach them (see also Chapter 12).

Here are some general guidelines:

• approach the person slowly in a calm and gentle manner

• speak normally but allow them time to understand

• give the person lots of reassurance

• try to gain the person's trust before carrying out any procedures with them

• always explain what you need to do and why

• show the person any equipment you are going to use, and allow them time to ask questions

• try to remember that the person may feel bewildered or frightened and this may show itself as aggression or lack of co-operation.

Learning disabilities

People with learning disabilities (see Chapter 10) may grow physically at a normal rate, but their mental functioning, and sometimes their emotional functioning too, is delayed. Some people with learning disabilities do not reach the usual adult level of functioning and are sometimes described as having a mental age of five, ten or whatever.

It is important to try to find out more about the person from the staff with whom you work or from the person's friends or relatives. However general guidelines to assist communication are as follows:

• approach the person as an adult, if they are so in age

• speak in a normal voice but give one piece of information at a time and allow time for them to take in the information

• if the person is having difficulty in understanding, cut out all unnecessary detail and concentrate on conveying the important information

• give them plenty of reassurance and try to get to know them

• observe carefully the things that they seem to cope with and the things that they find difficult, so that you can try to speak to the person at the right level for their understanding

• the person may have difficulty in learning and remembering, so that they may need repetition and frequent reminders.

Children

Probably the most important point when talking to children is to have realistic expectations of what they can understand at their age. Most children begin to use words to ask for things at about two years of age, but you need to think about the way you speak to any child under five (see Chapter 8).

Just as parents will often make up games to help children eat or behave reasonably in the car on a long journey, the same kind of games can be used in carrying out routine care procedures.

By the age of five most children who are developing normally have a good grasp of language, speak clearly and have a large vocabulary. They can understand most of what is said to them but some aspects of language such as jokes and sarcasm are still too difficult for them. You can still hear immaturities in their speech, but the basic language system is working well and you should be able to understand them easily.

Some children do not develop speech and language for a number of reasons such as hearing deficits, learning difficulties (mental handicap), emotional difficulties, physical handicap and prolonged illness. It is likely that you will meet children with communication problems in the course of your work.

Listen to what the child can say and try to reply at that level. If you are speaking to a five year old child who says "want dolly", which is characteristic of language used by two to three year olds, then you may need to use simpler language when you are talking to them than you would normally use with a five year old.

Some children with physical handicaps such as cerebral palsy may not be able to speak at all but may have developed good understanding of language. Whenever you are unsure, ask the child's parents what their child can understand.

Some children find strangers and nursing care procedures very frightening and may not want to talk at all. Don't press the child to give you an answer but talk to them reassuringly. If the child's parents are not with the child, tell them that the child is being very quiet and obviously needs reassurance. But remember that even noisy children can be anxious.

Above all, remember that you probably already know how best to talk to a frightened or worried child. Most people who have children of their own, or young relatives, develop their own strategies which work very well!

Below is a list of medical problems that are likely to cause communication problems or disorder in children:

Hearing loss: Some children who are deaf from birth hear very little while other children develop ear infections which usually cause temporary hearing problems.

Head injury due to road traffic accidents, brain tumours, stroke: Head injury in children is unfortunately relatively common; strokes in children are rare but do happen. Any damage to the brain may cause temporary communication problems, but some children may have more long term speech and language problems.

Cerebral palsy and muscle diseases may cause difficulty in using the speech muscles and in producing intelligible speech. Feeding may also be affected.

Cleft lip and palate: children born with clefts of the lip and/or palate are likely to have feeding problems as babies. Usually operations to repair the lip and palate are carried out before the child is one year old, but some children need a succession of operations. These children are prone to problems with speech and may have hearing problems due to repeated ear infections.

Hearing problems

Do not shout at someone who has hearing problems. When you shout or even raise your voice, you distort the normal patterns of speech and make it more difficult for the person to hear you. If the person is a lip reader, shouting will distort your facial movements too.

The world is a very noisy place, but those of us with normal hearing can ignore it most of the time. However, a lot of background noise makes it much more difficult for someone with a hearing loss to hear, even if they wear a hearing aid.

Hearing aids

When a person uses a hearing aid it is important to check regularly that it is in full working order, and to ensure that it is **switched on** when needed. Models and types of hearing aids vary, but the following points are important:

• **Batteries**. These last between one and three months. When they run out they should be kept, and returned to the issuing audiology department where they can be exchanged for new ones free of charge. If the aid whistles when switched on, and with the volume turned up, the battery is charged. If you cannot get a whistle, it is dead. Batteries should be checked every week and every day if the person is confused.

• **Volume**. To find the best volume setting, adjust the volume to the point just below where a whistle is heard. Check the whistle

> **Speaking to a person with hearing difficulty:**
> • **face the person**
> • **speak clearly, do not shout**
> • **repeat exactly what you said if they look puzzled, so that your lip movements are also repeated**

does not return if the person shakes their head. Observe the person to see if they seem comfortable with this volume.

• **Plastic tube**. The sound passes through this tube, so it must be kept clean, free of wax and flexible. It should be renewed regularly at the audiology clinic.

• **Ear mould**. This is made for the individual, and cannot be worn by anyone else. The small hole at the end is where the sound enters the ear. If it becomes blocked with wax, the aid is much less efficient.

It is therefore essential that the person's ears are checked for wax every six months. Care staff should check and remove any wax obvious in the *outer* ear every day.

You may need to use a quiet room or office if you are giving the person important information and want to make sure they have heard. Sometimes it may be necessary to write your message down.

Before you talk to someone who has a hearing loss, do switch off any nearby radios or TV.

You may come across a very useful communication aid consisting of a microphone, into which you speak, connected to an amplifier which the person holds to their better ear. This type of hearing aid is sometimes more useful than a conventional hearing aid because it does not pick up the same amount of background noise.

Communication aids

Both adults and children who have long term communication problems may have a communication aid. Sometimes the aid is a portable computer or a similar electronic device which has a screen and some form of print-out. When you have spoken to the person, give them time to use the communication aid and look at the screen for their answer. Remember to speak to the person and not the screen!

Speech and language therapy

Speech and language therapists (formerly called speech therapists) provide a service to people with communication impairments or swallowing disorders. Anyone who has difficulty understanding, whose speech is not clear, or who has reading or writing problems may benefit from this service. Most community health services have departments to whom patients may be referred. Speech and language therapists will assess someone referred to them, give advice to staff, other carers and family and, where appropriate and possible, they will treat the problem.

Sometimes people are not referred for therapy if they have no speech, but speech and language therapists also help the speechless, sometimes by providing a communication aid for the person. On the other hand, sometimes after a stroke, a person may be speaking quite well but have difficulties reading or writing which the therapist may also be able to help.

If you think someone has a communication problem or swallowing disorder, you can ask for them to be referred to your local department.

Points to remember

Being a good communicator involves much more than just hearing accurately and speaking clearly. It involves establishing a rapport with the person by making them feel that you are really listening. So:
1. Establish appropriate posture and position, such as facing someone and perhaps sitting or kneeling to be at their level.
2. Look at the person. Gain eye contact.
3. Show that you are interested by listening carefully, nodding appropriately, and responding to what the person says.
4. Use a gesture such as touching their arm for reassurance, where appropriate.
5. Speak in a way that makes the person feel that what they want or are asking about is considered important.
6. Encourage people to talk about themselves, but also about more neutral topics such as the weather, or what has been happening in the news, or their family.
7. Maintain politeness and do not invade a person's privacy. Remember that people may have different views from you on what is appropriate for conversation.

NVQ Levels 2 & 3 Core Units
O Promote equality for all individuals.
U4 Contribute to the health, safety and security of individuals and their environment.
U5 Obtain, transmit and store information relating to the delivery of a care service.
Level 2 Core Unit
W2 Contribute to the ongoing support of clients and others significant to them.
Level 3 Core Unit
Z4 Promote communication where there are communication difficulties.
Z8 Support clients when they are distressed.
Y2 Enable clients to make use of available services and information.
Level 2 Direct care
Z6 Enable clients to maintain and improve their mobility.
Level 2 Domiciliary support
W8 Enable clients to maintain contacts in potentially isolating situations.

CHAPTER 6

Blind and partially sighted people

Rose Ashbee

- *How to help and communicate with blind and partially sighted people*
- *Sign languages • Guiding, and safety in the environment*

When you approach a blind or partially sighted person, always introduce yourself, say who you are and what your job is. Do stop and chat if you have the time, and always say what you are doing. Address each individual by name – after all, they cannot see that you are talking to them. Never leave without saying goodbye: it is frustrating and embarrassing for a person to realise that they are talking to an empty space. Do not shout: many sight impaired people have excellent hearing. Speak clearly and at a normal pitch.

How easily someone who is deaf and blind can communicate depends on several factors. Firstly, how old they were when they lost their sight and hearing, secondly whether they lost both senses at once or one after another and thirdly whether they have learned a language beforehand, either speech or sign.

Language and speech are not the same thing. Language is the ability to understand and communicate information. Speech is one method of doing this, gesture and touch are others.

People whose first handicap was deafness may know British sign language and finger spelling. They should not find it too difficult to use the deaf blind manual alphabet, as it is an adaptation of the deaf manual spelled out on the hand. An alternative is the Spartan alphabet, block capitals printed on the hand.

If the individual has enough sight you may try using a thick, black felt tipped pen and writing (on paper) in large print. Whatever method you choose, you must use it consistently. It is best to start off by linking it to essential information about some activity, such as meals, dressing or bathing.

When visiting a partially sighted person at home, always encourage them to use a door chain. Explain to them who you are and why you are visiting. If you carry an identification card, hand it to them so that they can examine it closely.

Let them touch

When you approach someone who is deaf and blind let them know you are there without startling them, by tapping them gently on the forearm or wrist. To make sure they know who you are, let them feel a ring or a badge or a hair slide that you always wear. Or make an agreed movement on their hand such as touching their palm gently.

Don't be put off if a deaf and blind person wants to use touch; remember it is the most important information sense they have left. Do use every opportunity to communicate and involve them in what is going on around them.

Guiding

Do ask first if a person wants assistance: no one likes to be grabbed and dragged. Let the person take your arm and walk slightly in front of them, watching out carefully for obstacles. If you need to walk in single file, through an open doorway for example, indicate this by tucking your guiding hand behind your back.

Always stop at the beginning of stairs and steps and say whether they are going up or down and about how many there are. If there is a handrail put the person's hand on it to help them. Make sure you say when you have reached the last step.

Help the sight impaired person to sit down by putting their hand on the back of the chair. Leave the rest to them; never lower them bodily into a chair they have not inspected.

Mealtimes

Always ask what an individual likes and dislikes. There is nothing worse than putting an item of food into your mouth that you dislike. When serving a meal do remember to say that you have done so. Say what it is and the position it occupies on the plate and stick to the same system. For example, always place meat at 12 o'clock, potatoes at 6 o'clock and vegetables at 3 and 9 o'clock.

Do ask if help is needed, perhaps by cutting up the food. Providing a plate with an upturned rim will assist the sight-impaired person to feed themselves and reduce the risk and embarrassment of

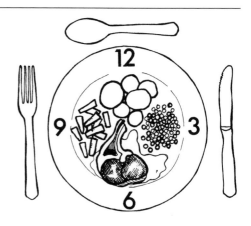

It helps to use the idea of a clock face to describe a plate of food to a blind person.

food sliding onto the table. When serving drinks say where you are placing them, and never over-fill cups or glasses; this will reduce the risk of spillage.

Dressing

Just because a person cannot see how they look does not mean to say that they do not want to look nice. Never let a sight impaired person go about with odd coloured shoes on, laddered stockings, untidy hair or grubby clothing. They will rely on you to tell them tactfully if anything is amiss.

The environment

Even people registered as blind may have some degree of sight. This does not mean that they are able to "see", but they may perhaps be able to distinguish between light and dark. Visual handicaps are so variable and the conditions that enable people to make the best use of their eyesight may vary considerably. Always make sure the individual knows where the light switches are.

Make sure they know how to get to the

bathroom, lavatory, day room and dining area in an unfamiliar environment. Try to mention easy to touch landmarks, such as pictures on the wall, or a change in surface from carpet to tiling underfoot. Watch out for hazards in their path such as hoovers, commodes, trailing flexes or tea trolleys. Always say if you have to leave something in the way, or if something must not be touched. If you move anything always put it back exactly in the same place.

Never put a sight-impaired person's belongings away before asking where they should go.

A little extra help

Do not worry about saying things like "Do you see what I mean?". Avoiding this can often create more difficulties for everyone if a silence follows while you search for a different word.

Be natural. Your tone of voice and your manner is vitally important; it must convey what you intend it to. Sight-impaired people cannot see your face, whether you are smiling, worried or cross. Do not be afraid to touch. A friendly pat on the back or a squeeze of the hand can be reassuring and comforting.

But the greatest need for most deaf or blind people is for companionship. Someone to talk to them at their own pace. To tell them what is going on in the world outside. Remember that sight-impaired people are normal people who just can't see. Treat them as you would treat anyone else, except at those times when they need a little extra help. Just as you would in their place.

Points to remember

1. Address each individual by name and always introduce yourself. Stay and chat if you have time, and never leave without saying goodbye.
2. Don't be put off if a deaf and blind person wants to use touch.
3. Ask if someone wants assistance – never grab and drag.
4. At mealtimes, special help is needed.
5. Don't let people go about looking grubby or untidy.
6. Make sure they know how to get to the bathroom, lavatory and dining area.
7. Watch out for hazards and tell blind people about them.
8. Remember that their greatest need is for companionship.

Resources

National Deaf Blind Helpers League, 18 Rainbow Court, Paston Ridings, Peterborough PE4 6UP. Tel: 0733 73511. Information, advice and publications, including illustrated instructions for manual alphabets.

Royal National Institute for the Blind, 224 Great Portland St, London W1N 6AA. Advice, information and publications, especially Braille books, periodicals and music, and Moon books and periodicals.

NVQ Levels 2 & 3 Core Units

O Promote equality for all individuals

U4 Contribute to the health, safety and security of individuals and their environment.

U5 Obtain, transmit and store information relating to the delivery of a care service.

Level 2 Core Unit

W2 Contribute to the ongoing support of clients and others significant to them.

Level 2 Direct Care

Z9 Enable clients to maintain their personal hygiene and appearance.

Z10 Enable clients to eat and drink.

Z11 Enable clients to access and use toilet facilities.

Z19 Enable clients to achieve physical comfort.

Level 2 Domiciliary support

W8 Enable clients to maintain contacts in potentially isolating situations.

U1 Contribute to the maintenance and management of domestic and personal resources.

Level 3 Core Unit

Z4 Promote communication where there are communication difficulties.

Y2 Enable clients to make use of available services and information.

CHAPTER 7

Promoting and educating for health

Liz Day

• Definitions of health • Valuing what you do • The family's health • Seeking advice • Preventing problems • Health of the Nation • Accident prevention

In your work as a care assistant you are expected to promote good health – but what does this mean? Health means very different things to different individuals. Standard "healthy living" advice will not do; an individual approach is needed. Some important things to think about are set out in this chapter, to give you some guidance and food for thought.

Definitions of health

Health is a word which is used a great deal and we often assume that everyone is talking about the same thing. If you think about some of the different ways in which the word "health" appears, you will see what I mean. There are health foods, health farms, health shops, health centres, the National Health Service, health and fitness suites, the Health of the Nation, "Cheers – Good Health" (a toast with alcohol!) to name just a few. You can probably think of other such words and titles in common use.

The words "health foods", imply that if you buy certain foods from health shops, health will be assured. You can also go to a health farm or a health centre and obtain health. But a health farm will provide a completely different service to that which may be obtained at a health centre. At a health farm, the customer will probably have a programme of activity, rest and special diet, which will improve the customer's wellbeing. On the other hand, if the same customer goes to a health centre, they may undergo a procedure such as a cervical smear, a tetanus injection or ear syringing, or they could see a doctor and and receive advice, have a diagnosis made and treatment started.

It may seem very obvious to you that different types of services are available in the different centres. The point is that the word "health" is used in both services yet what is actually available is very different.

What is health?

You may want to stop and consider for a few minutes, what it means to you to be healthy.

You may think that being physically fit, active and free from illness is health. You may think that peace of mind, having good relationships, a clean environment, fresh air, shelter, warmth and food is good health. Although there are numerous definitions of health, it is a very personal state and even though some people have a health problem, they may feel healthy because they are able to do what they want to do within their limitations and with the love and the support of others.

It helps to think of health as having seven dimensions: physical, mental, social, emotional, spiritual, environmental and societal. Our feeling of wellbeing may be affected in any of these dimensions. Here are some examples of the way in which different people may respond to an event which affects their health.

If an individual measures their health in physical terms – such as someone who goes jogging or does aerobics regularly – and they experience a health problem such as a painful knee or back, they may feel very unwell if they cannot undertake their preferred activity. Someone who has experienced a bereavement may feel physically ill and have very real symptoms, although their main problem is coping with loss.

Someone who is unable to practise their faith because of lack of sensitivity or opportunity, may feel unwell and unhappy. An individual who loses their faithful pet, may feel unwell as a result of this bereavement. Someone who feels afraid to go out for fear of racist abuse may feel psychologically unwell.

It takes sensitivity and good communication skills to be able to deal with these important influences on the health of individuals.

Valuing what you do

It is important to recognise and value the activities which people undertake to promote their own health. It is very easy to identify what people "should" or "ought" to do to stay healthy. We all know roughly what we need to do to be healthy in terms of taking exercise, not smoking, eating the "right" foods etc. These health messages seem to bombard us from the pages of newspapers, magazines and journals. They seem to ignore the actions which we actually do undertake. This is a criticism which may also be directed at health promoters.

Jot down some of things which you do or which you think are important to do to maintain and improve your health. Check your list against the list below which is in no particular order of priority.

Self-health promotion activities
• Eat a good diet
• Drink adequate fluids
• Limit the intake of alcohol
• Clean your teeth regularly
• Reduce or give up smoking
• Go to the dentist
• Attend the optician regularly
• Take regular exercise
• Have regular screening tests
• Keep warm/cool
• Wash regularly
• Treat minor injuries
• Have immunisations/vaccines
• Sleep and rest
• Take care with prescribed medicines
• Get advice on over-the-counter drugs
• Relax and enjoy yourself
• Confide in a friend
• Express your emotions (cry, get cross)
• Regulate weight
• Drive carefully
• Wear seatbelts
• Take care of your pets
• Wash your hands before eating
• Take care when lifting
• Wear well fitting shoes
• Mental stimulation
• Practice your religion
• Regulate pregnancy
• Practice safe sex
• Participate in relationships
• Work

You have probably listed other actions which do not appear on this list (it is not exclusive). You will see that these activities

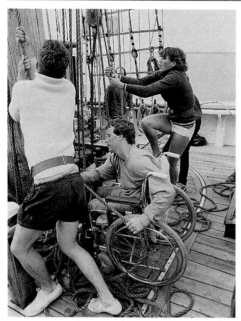

Health means different things to different individuals. Find out what people do to promote their own health, and build on these strategies.

of professionals) to say nothing of well meaning relatives and friends. Each will be able to give some advice on the best ways of carrying out care.

The physiotherapist may say that in addition to all the tasks which the family is already undertaking there is a need for a specified period of exercise each day. The speech therapist advises some speech exercises and the dentist advises brushing and flossing of teeth. When the various therapies and treatments are added up, there may be little time for the pleasurable things in life, and the family may be left with a feeling of not being able to do enough for the child, and that their own needs do not count at all.

The health of the whole family needs to be taken into account as well as individual needs. It may be more important that they are able to have time and space for themselves as individuals than it is to carry out certain activities which could be undertaken by a paid carer or a volunteer.

include the seven different dimensions of health, yet the key message from health promoters tends to focus on those areas which play only a minor part in our overall wellbeing, the physical dimension, and rarely focuses on all the things we are already doing.

The whole family's health

When you stop and think about a particular situation, such as the family that has a child with special needs who is dependent upon the family members for all aspects of personal hygiene, dressing, activity, eating and drinking, the family may feel under pressure if professionals have unrealistic expectations of what they "should" do for the child.

The child may be seen by a physiotherapist, doctor, speech therapist, dentist, nurse and teacher (just a few of the army

Seeking advice

It may also be assumed that when someone is concerned about their health, the first person to whom they turn is someone in the health service, but in reality, this may not be the case.

Think back to the last time you were concerned about your health or when you felt unwell. What did you do? Jot down some of the actions which you took and compare them with the list below.

Depending on the urgency of the situation you may have done a number of things. You may have told someone with whom you could confide, the symptoms you were experiencing and they may have suggested you "wait and see", "have a day off", "take some tablets", "see your medical adviser", (who incidentally could be a hakim or herbalist and not necessarily a doctor of Western medicine). It may have been suggested by your friend/partner that you see the doctor.

Your actions may be determined by a number of things such as your past experience with the symptoms and the way in which your concerns were dealt with by the doctor. They may be determined by your response to over-the-counter drugs or the reactions of colleagues and superiors when you take a day off for ill health reasons.

An elderly person may feel that there is no point in seeking medical advice, if they have previously been told "It's your age", and their concerns have not been taken seriously. Health education may enable them to argue from a position of strength if they have more knowledge about what normal ageing means in physical terms.

It is very important to find out what people do to promote their own health, what they do if they are not feeling too well, and to build on these strategies, rather than ignore or discredit them.

Having looked at what people already do to promote their own health, let us now turn to the ways in which health may be promoted and ill-health prevented. This is often referred to as primary, secondary and tertiary prevention.

Preventing problems

Health education may be provided to different clients in anticipation of a possible health problem. You may advise someone about eating the right foods and taking enough fluid even though they have no problems. The purpose of your advice is to ensure that they stay well, to improve healing and prevent infection. For example, enough fluid and fibre in the diet to prevent constipation, or foods rich in iron to prevent anaemia. This is called **primary prevention**. The aim is to prevent a problem occurring at all.

The client may complain of tiredness or feeling unwell; you may advise them to go to the doctor or see the nurse because you know that these feelings may be symptoms of an existing condition. The client may be taking some tablets for anaemia or for an infection. You may help them to understand the directions on the bottle so that they take them at the right time and in the right dose. This is called **secondary prevention** because you are seeking to find out if they already have something wrong or, if they have, that they take the necessary action to prevent it getting worse.

Secondary prevention also includes giving information to people about what to do if an accident or incident occurs. A nurse or doctor may give advice to a carer or parent so that they know what to do if a child has a febrile convulsion (a fit) as a result of a high temperature.

The client may have an existing condition such as arthritis which makes it difficult for them to move around, manage their housework, cook and care for themselves. Advising them of the different aids and appliances, helping them with rehabilitation and thus helping them to retain their independence, is called **tertiary prevention**. That is undertaking health promotion in order to prevent or reduce further deterioration in the client's health.

These three levels of health education are a vital part of all care work. Separating prevention in this way helps to distinguish different approaches to health education, but sometimes the three levels may be implemented with one client.

Think about a client who has multiple sclerosis. There may be quite a bit of preventive work being undertaken in terms of rehabilitation, providing aids and appliances, encouraging membership of a support group and generally maintaining current levels of health (tertiary prevention). The client may be a woman who needs cervical cytology, breast screening, vision, hearing and dental checks, and other health maintenance checks (secondary prevention). The client may also benefit from exercise for pleasure, immunisations, advice about diet, sex including safe sex, accident prevention, continence promotion and many other subjects (primary prevention). Some people associate primary prevention with children and tertiary prevention with older people or those who are ill. But everyone can benefit from health promotion and preventive activities at each of these important levels.

The Health of the Nation

In 1993 the Government published its policy document *Health of the Nation*. Five key targets have been set to reduce the number of premature deaths and unnecessary ill-health from specific conditions which are prevalent in our society. Deaths and ill-health caused by cancers, mental illness, coronary heart disease, sexually transmitted diseases including HIV/AIDS and accidents are the main targets identified in the policy.

If we now look at one of the targets, **accidents**, and one specific age group, **children**, it will be clear that the responsibility for preventing accidents and promoting a safe environment is shared by many different people at different levels in different organisations.

Accident prevention

Individuals and families

When prevention of accidents involving small children is examined, it is clear that parents play a key role in protecting them, ensuring that any equipment used in their care is properly maintained, that medicines are locked up and household cleaning fluids are carefully stored. It is also parents' responsibility to ensure that children have safe play things.

Local authorities

Local planning authorities and local councils play a part in preventing accidents by advising developers and architects about the use of glass in doors, the positioning of cooker spaces, the type of window frames and window catches used in family accomodation. The use of glass (safety glass) in doors is now controlled by the Building Regulations. Under the new safety regulations, architects will have more direct responsibility for safety.

Local councils may be responsible for the provision of children's playgrounds and the equipment such as swings and slides. They are responsible for the inspection and registration of playgroups and nurseries and play a part in the appointment of staff.

Manufacturers

Manufacturers will need to ensure that play equipment is of the safest possible design. The council will need to ensure that it is placed on surfaces which can minimise the effects of a fall, and that it is inspected and maintained regularly. Manufacturers will also need to ensure that all equipment and toys are made to the highest possible safety standards to reduce the possibility of accidents occuring as a result of using that equipment.

Government

The government is responsible for introducing legislation which also protects children including seat belt laws, safety standards for design and manufacture of equipment.

Pharmacists

Pharmacists are responsible for ensuring that medication is provided in the proper containers with childproof caps. The problem with these is that sometimes adults with arthritis or who have had a stroke, find it difficult to open them too!

Voluntary organisations

Voluntary organisations such as the Child Accident Prevention Trust can play an important part by undertaking research with parents and professionals and providing up-to-date advice and health promotional materials for them.

Health services

Accident and emergency departments have a responsibility to provide prompt and appropriate treatment for any children who have been unfortunate enough to be involved in an accident. The hospital services may also need to provide rehabilitation and after care if it is needed in order to help the child to recover to as near as possible their previous level of functioning prior to the accident.

All community care staff have a part to play in advising parents about safety precautions such as the use of fire and radiator guards, the safe storage of drugs, the use of stair gates, cooker and socket guards. Advice may also be given about children's developmental stages and particular risks, so that they may anticipate potential risks and plan accordingly. Of course all accidents cannot be prevented, but they can be reduced. (See chapter 14, Safety and First Aid.)

Whether you work in the local clinic, surgery or in the home, you will need to know the safety needs of children and their families and should be able to give up to date advice on preventive measures.

Using accidents and small children as one example, it is clear that the responsibility for health promotion and health education is not just the responsibility of parents but is the responsibility of different organisations and at all levels including individual, local community, health services, governments, manufacturers and voluntary levels. We all have a part to play in this important activity.

1 Activity:
Health of the Nation targets

Think about one of the other Health of the Nation health targets, such as mental health, cancers, coronary heart disesase or sexually transmitted disease and jot down the responsibilities of as many of these key levels and organisations as you can. When you have completed your notes, share them with your team leader and discuss them so that you can develop a comprehensive understanding of these levels particularily in your area of work. You might like to compare your notes on HIV/AIDs with the example provided below.

Comments: HIV/AIDS and Sexual Health

Individuals and families

When considering the prevention of HIV/AIDS and the promotion of sexual health, it could be argued that individuals are responsible for their own actions. But as with the prevention of accidents, it can be seen that the different levels of different organisations have a responsibility to promote sexual health too.

Adults are responsible for protecting themselves and others from unwanted pregnancies and from sexually transmitted diseases. They may do this by utilising effective family planning methods, limiting their sexual partners and by using condoms when engaged in penetrative sexual activity.

Family members have a responsibility for the education of their children about sexuality, sexual health and safe sex.

You have the same responsibilities as other members of society in promoting your own sexual health.

Local authorities

You may wonder how local authorities could be responsible for the promotion of sexual health and the prevention of HIV/AIDS. Local authorities are responsible for local education and the implementation of the National Curriculum in schools. It will, through the teaching staff, ensure that personal and social education is provided which will include the fostering of self esteem, self awareness and moral values and issues.

In-service training will also enable teachers to further develop their skills in dealing with sensitive and controversial issues which often arise as a result of open and honest discussions. Teachers will also need to work within the local policies and guidelines on dealing with accidents, first aid and blood spillage in school.

Manufacturers

Manufacturers will need to ensure that their products such as condoms are readily available through vending machines and through other retail outlets. They will need to ensure that their products are reliable and conform to British Standards and that any information they give is clear and unambiguous.

Government

The Government will need to provide clear guidelines about the importing of blood products and to undertake quality assurance measures and auditing to ensure that the guidelines are being adhered to.

The Government also funds the Health Education Authority and may be involved in specific health education campaigns. It has also been responsible for the development and publication of the *Health of the Nation* policy document and associated handbooks (primary prevention).

Government will need to provide expert advice on dealing with blood products, advice to staff such as surgeons and dentists about dealing with clients who are HIV positive, or if the surgeons or dentists are HIV positive (secondary prevention).

It will also be responsible for the provision of specialist centres to help people affected by HIV/AIDS and other sexually transmitted diseases (tertiary prevention).

Pharmacists

Pharmacists may be able to provide advice and information as well as specific products such as condoms. This advice could include information on the unwanted side effects of drugs or medical conditions such as diabetes, which may produce impotence. Pharmacists may be able to advise or they may suggest that clients discuss it with a nurse or general practitioner, if they do not have the facilities for confidential discussion.

They may also sell pregnancy testing equipment and be able to advise on its use.

Voluntary organisations

Youth clubs, guides and scout groups may be responsible for educating about health including sexual health and family planning. They may be responsible for teaching first aid which would include the prevention of the spread of HIV/AIDS when giving first aid (primary prevention).

There are a number of important voluntary organisations which are involved in secondary and tertiary prevention. They provide helplines, guidance and support which is so essential for people who may have a need for advice about pregnancy, termination of pregnancy or when they have been diagnosed as being HIV positive. (See resource list, especially *Health of the Nation* Key Area Handbooks.)

Health services

The services available through the NHS are numerous. They include general practitioners, family planning nurses, school nurses, practice nurses, midwives, health visitors, district nurses, community mental handicap nurses, community psychiatric nurses, and HIV coordinators. These different members of the community health care teams may provide drop-in centres, preconceptual care, immunisation including rubella screening and immunisation, cervical screening clinics, well person clinics, health promotion days. These activities are primary and secondary prevention. Tertiary prevention includes the provision of genito-urinary management clinics, and psychosexual counselling.

You should also be given the opportunity for regular updating and in-service training to enable you to play your part effectively in sexual health promotion and the prevention of HIV/AIDS. Being aware of the range of services available in the community and being able to advise clients on how to use the services, is an important part of health promotion.

Briefly return to the earlier section on accident prevention and children and see if you can identify those activities and measures taken by different organisations, which fall into primary, secondary and tertiary prevention categories.

2 Activity:
Mr and Mrs Stevens

Look at the following case study and think about the advantages of health promotion. Try to organise your ideas of health promotion with this couple, into primary, secondary and tertiary prevention.

Mr and Mrs Stevens live in a three bedroomed semi-detached house. They are in their early seventies, and their children are now married and have moved away. The children do keep in regular contact and visit when they can.

Mr Stevens has dementia and as long as he continues in his usual routines, he functions reasonably well with support and supervision from his wife. He likes to potter in the garden although he can only dig and weed and occasionally pulls plants up by mistake.

He loves walking and he and his wife walk about five miles every afternoon.

They like to attend the local church together although Mr Stevens forgets that he has been soon after attending. They live on a small private pension and the state pension so they are not financially very secure.

He needs help with dressing and undressing. He would get lost if he went out walking on his own. He gets very restless if he is unable to go for his walk, if the weather is bad for example.

Mrs Stevens is two years younger than her husband. She is generally fit and well although she does need surgery for a gynaecological problem. She is very concerned about her husband. She enjoys gardening, walking and socialising. She is unable to attend the local Women's Institute (WI) now because she cannot leave her husband. She enjoys swimming and used to go at least once a week but has had to give this up too.

In what ways would it be possible to promote the health and wellbeing of Mr and Mrs Stevens?

Comment: Mr and Mrs Stevens

Mrs Stevens
Primary prevention

Mrs Stevens may need someone who will look after her husband while she has a swim once a week, and while she attends her local WI. These two activities help her with physical health and her social and emotional health.

She may have friends with whom she may be able to confide when she goes to these activities, which may be very important for her mental health. She should be immunised against tetanus (as she is a gardener) and against influenza.

Mrs Stevens needs some advice regarding financial benefits which she could claim as she is providing 24-hour care for her husband. She might also welcome some advice about local services which could provide some respite from this full-time commitment.

Mrs Stevens might benefit from joining a local carers group or a group for carers of people with Alzheimer's disease and dementias.

Secondary prevention

Mrs Stevens may need a dietary supplement of iron if she has a gynaecological problem requiring surgery, as she may have developed anaemia.

Tertiary prevention

She may need help with the gardening, housework and care of her husband while she has surgery and recovers from it. Her anxiety would be greatly relieved if she knew that someone would come and stay in her house and care for her husband while she is in hospital.

Mr Stevens

Primary prevention

Although Mr Stevens has dementia, he enjoys his daily walks, he likes gardening and is very mobile. He needs a partner to walk with him for company and to prevent him from either losing his way or from having an accident.

He should also be immunised against tetanus. He may also benefit from influenza vaccine in the autumn. He will need to be encouraged and helped to maintain a good level of nutrition and adequate fluids to keep him in good health.

Secondary prevention

Mr Stevens may need to have his ears checked for wax as he may not be able to complain about any hearing difficulties. He may need vision, hearing and dental checks to keep him in good health. The practice nurse running Well Person Clinics at their doctor's surgery may be able to offer Mr Stevens a screening service which will detect health problems, and will be able to refer him to his general practitioner if necessary.

Tertiary prevention

Mr Stevens has dementia but he is also fit and well. Helping him continue in his usual and preferred routines may help to keep him in closer touch with his reality.

You will probably identify some other ideas for health promotion with this couple. You could discuss this case study with the practice nurse to determine the contribution which could be made to the health of this couple.

When you consider the seven dimensions of health which were mentioned earlier, you will appreciate that as well as promoting the physical well-being of the couple, you would also be promoting their **social, emotional and mental health.**

They continue to maintain their **spiritual health** as they are able to attend their church. The church could also provide practical and emotional support.

Environmental health is promoted through a range of measures including the monitoring of air and water supplies, inspection of supermarkets and the collection of refuse. **Societal health** is measured by the care society provides for its vulnerable citizens.

When considering the other *Health of the Nation* targets, it is clear in looking at this small case study that you could be contributing to the achievement of the targets associated with mental health, cancer and coronary heart disease prevention.

The promotion of the three dimensions of mental, social and psychological health are a particularily important contribution to the mental health target. Enabling Mrs Stevens to relinquish her caring role from time to time, enabling her to maintain her contacts with friends and confidantes or attend a carers group may promote her mental health by relieving the stress which she must experience. Encouraging them to continue their mutual physical activities and Mrs Stevens to continue her swimming may contribute to the prevention of coronary heart disease. Maintaining mobility may play an important part in

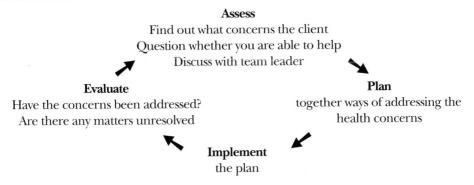

Assess
Find out what concerns the client
Question whether you are able to help
Discuss with team leader

Evaluate
Have the concerns been addressed?
Are there any matters unresolved

Plan
together ways of addressing the
health concerns

Implement
the plan

Fig 1. A Problem-solving cycle for health promotion.

preventing accidents as good posture, strong muscles and stamina will prevent falls.

Working with the practice nurse and encouraging the Stevens to take up the screening services may contribute to the prevention of cancers.

So while we have examined two of the health targets in detail and identified the importance of a multi-agency approach to the achievement of the targets, we have also, through the exploration of a case-study, identified ways in which each of the targets may be promoted with one family.

The Health Promotion Cycle

Having had the opportunity to look at Mr and Mrs Stevens, you have seen that there are a number of ways in which they promote their own health and the possible opportunities for you to contribute to their health promotion.

When you are visiting clients it is important to appreciate some of the possible ways in which you may promote their well-being, but it is also very important that you find out what health concerns they have which would benefit from health education and health promotion.

When considering ways in which you can promote the health of clients like Mr and Mrs Stevens, it is useful to do so in a systematic way. This may be approached using a problem-solving cycle (Fig 1).

Assessment

The **first** and most important aspect of health promotion is to find out and assess what the client's main health concerns may be. They may feel that they do not get enough exercise, that they eat too much food containing fats, sugar, salt or not enough fibre. They may feel very stressed because they are caring for someone who is not in good health or because their caring role isolates them from other people in a similar situation. They may need advice about family planning and safe sex or find it difficult to know how to discipline their children.

When clients have identified their concerns, it is important to reflect on your own knowledge of those and other health concerns. If you do not have up-to-date information about the concerns, you do need to find out from the client whether or not they mind if you seek advice from your team leader. Confidentiality is very important and guidelines need to be discussed with your team leader so that you have a clear idea about the areas which you are expected to refer back and discuss, and those areas in which you and the client may reach agreement in confidence.

This stage in the process may include learning more about the subject yourself so that you may give accurate and up-to-date information. This may be especially important if the client is unable to go out. You can share the information with them, giving them copies of the articles which you have found useful.

Planning

The **second** stage is to plan together the best ways to address the health concerns. It may be that your client is able to go out. If this is the case the client may like to meet someone in a similar situation, or to visit the local library and find the information for themselves. If the client has a health need or concern which requires a more in-depth discussion, your team leader may undertake a visit with you or on their own, or may ask another professional to undertake a visit, depending on the sensitivity of the subject or issue.

This stage includes setting realistic goals which are possible to evaluate. For example, if the client wanted to take more exercise, you may have agreed that they take a 10 minute walk every other day, or instead of using the remote control on the television, they get out of the chair and change the programme by hand. You may agree to find out more about pain relief and arthritis from your team leader and from the Arthritis and Rheumatism Council (see resource list) within one week. It is always useful to make a deadline date, otherwise plans tend to drift.

Implementation

The **third** stage is that of implementation, carrying out what was agreed in the previous stage. You can see that if the goals were realistic both you and the client will have a clear idea of what each of you has to do.

Evaluation

The **fourth**, and note not the final stage, is that of evaluation. How are you both progressing with your goals. Have they been achieved? What problems have been encountered? Have they addressed the concerns of the client or has anything else happened in their life which has changed their priorities?

You will realise from the sort of questions which could be asked at the evaluation stage, that health promotion is not a static situation but one which is dynamic, constantly changing to meet the changing needs of clients. The answers which emerge will form part of the next stage, back to stage one (the assessment stage) thus completing a cycle.

This cycle may help you to identify needs which may be addressed through putting the client in touch with local relevant organisations, for support, for advice, for sharing ideas, for putting pressure on different organisations to change. People with small children or people who have mobility problems may, for example, want a safe crossing point to get from one side of the road to another close to the doctor's surgery, the shops or the bus stop. Helping people with similar concerns meet each other may bring about change.

These initiatives arising from initial assessment of their health concerns and needs should be evaluated, as well as more personal changes in lifestyle.

One of the major influences on health assessments arises from the assessor's own attitudes and values, which may be different from those of the client. It is important for those undertaking health promotion to be aware of their own attitudes and values as they can have a profound effect on the care that is given.

As mentioned earlier some people have negative views and low expectations of health in old age and may therefore fail to treat health problems as seriously as they might if it was a younger person experiencing the same health problems. Depression, for example, may be ignored or not even detected in an older person, but may receive serious consideration, counselling, support, medication and other interventions if the person is much younger.

People who smoke, drink, are obese, or lead "risky" lifestyles may also be unfairly judged especially if they have a health problem which is associated with that lifestyle. You may like to consider some of the reasons which you have heard for unfair judgements being made and also consider how these can be overcome.

Points to remember

1. Each of us has an important part to play in health promotion, either in promoting our own health or the health of others.

2. Health is not a simple concept: we all have different ideas about what affects our health.

3. Different organisations play an important part through their interventions and actions to promote different dimensions of health. A concerted effort is needed by people at all levels of responsibility if each of the Government's *Health of the Nation* targets is to be achieved.

4. There are different levels of health promotion directed towards primary, secondary and tertiary prevention. Even if an older client has a chronic health problem such as dementia, primary prevention is possible.

5. In a problem solving approach to health promotion, it is important to work in partnership with the client, to meet their goals and their concerns.

6. Assessment, planning, implementation and evaluation of health promotion should be a process shared with the client.

7. Your role in health promotion in the community may include putting people in touch with relevant local organisations for further support and advice.

8. The aim of health promotion is helping people to change their lifestyle within their culture, values and beliefs. It may also be directed at getting organisations such as the Health Service and governments, local and national, to make changes in order to meet the health needs of local people and communities.

9. Local communities have an important partnership role in working with health care professionals to influence change. You will be part of the process both as an individual and within the local community.

Further reading

Calnan M (1987) *Health and Illness. The Lay Perspective.* Tavistock, London and New York

Department of Health (1993) *Health of the Nation.* HMSO, London.

Department of Health (1993) Key Area Handbooks on **Health of the Nation Targets**. HMSO, London.

Ewles L, Simnett I (1992) *Promoting Health. A Practical Guide.* Scutari, London.

Hubley J (1993) *Communicating Health.* Macmillan, London.

The Health Education Authority is a good source of materials which will be useful to you and to your clients. You may send for leaflets such as: *Changing What You Eat, Resources for patients and primary health care professionals.* These and many other resources may also be available from your local health promotion department. See also Useful Addresses on p187.

Copies of the Health of the Nation Key Area Handbooks are available free from: BAPS, Health Publication Unit Heywood Stores No 2 Site, Manchester Road Heywood Lancashire OL10 2PZ.

NVQ Levels 2 & 3 Core Units
O Promote equality for all individuals.
U4 Contribute to the health, safety and security of individuals and their environment.
U5 Obtain, transmit and store information relating to the delivery of a care service.

Level 2 Core Unit
W2 Contribute to the ongoing support of clients and others significant to them.

Level 3 Core Unit
Z8 Support clients when they are distressed.
Y2 Enable clients to make use of available services and information.

Level 2 Direct Care
Z10 Enable clients to eat and drink.
Z11 Enable clients to access and use toilet facilities.

Level 2 Domiciliary Support
W8 Enable clients to maintain contacts in potentially isolating situations.

CHAPTER 8
Keeping children healthy

Jo Carroll and Louise Hembrough

• Child health• Child development • Physical health
• Psychological health • Child health surveillance • Measuring sight
and hearing • Immunisations • Teenagers

Good physical and psychological health in childhood is essential for normal growth and development and for shaping future generations. A knowledge of the way in which children grow and develop is important to understand how things may go wrong or why illness may occur in later life.

Many health, social service and education workers are involved in promoting healthy or "normal" child development. It is also important that the health and well-being of parents is safeguarded by providing information and support. Leaflets are designed by the Health Education Authority for parents and you may wish to ensure that these are available in your workplace.

As a health care assistant, you may be required to help a health visitor, school nurse or doctor to monitor and record aspects of child health and development.

Table 1 – Developmental Stages

6-8 weeks Watches and follows faces, turns to the light, startled by loud noises.

3 months Wriggles and kicks, notices people and playthings, watches their own hands.

5 months Rolls over from back to front and front to back. Reaches for objects and grasps. Puts objects in mouth.

7/8 months Knows items exist when they are out of sight.

8 months Crawls, manipulates by opening and shutting, pushing, pulling, biting, twisting. Sits unaided, babbles ba-ba, da-da etc.

9 months Thumb and finger grips. Able to pull up to stand.

10 months Walks, holding onto furniture and objects

13 months Walks unaided, Crawls upstairs. Can do switches, knobs, dials. Interested in hidden objects.

18 months Imitates others when playing. Climbs furniture and objects, likes to empty and fill containers.

2 years Fascinated by smell, taste and textures.

3 years Uses potty or toilet. Understands what is said. Stops putting objects into mouth.

Preschool Climbs trees and other apparatus, runs and can use scissors.

Table 1 outlines child development at the major life stages. The table may help you to consider what a child should be doing at a certain age, the risks of accidents and the types of play activity that would be most appropriate.

As children develop, they learn new skills – how to speak, walk, gain attention and how to hold and manipulate various objects. It is important that children learn to adapt such skills. This will enable them to use cups and cutlery independently, to use the toilet when appropriate and to recognise the presence and individual needs of other children and adults around them. These changes develop from physical growth and because of stimulation and play with parents and other children.

Physical health

Food

Breast milk is the best food for babies. It is cheaper, easier than having to buy and sterilise bottles, and has all the natural vital nutrients that a child may need. Breast feeding is not always easy for some women and you may need to support a mother who has difficulty. Remember that any advice, help or support you give should support that given by the midwife, and not be based on your own ideas or experience.

There are a number of instant formula (powdered) milks available. Many mothers will use the milk recommended by the midwife or by friends. It is important that all equipment and bottles are clean and sterilised before use. Formula feeds must be made up to the correct strength, without extra sugar or anything else, and according to manufacturers' instructions.

Breast and formula milks are sufficient for babies up to three months of age, when it is recommended that a mixed diet (solids) is introduced. Some health professionals recommend that vitamin drops are also given to children.

Dental care

Parents are the best educators of dental care in young children. Encouraging regular brushing as soon as teeth erupt, and low sugar diets, will help to prevent damage to new teeth. Fluoride is added to water supplies in many parts of the country. Parents may also be advised to use fluoride drops by some health professionals.

Cleaning teeth should be encouraged after every meal and in the morning and evening. A pea-sized amount of a fluoride toothpaste with an appropriately sized toothbrush is generally recommended. Toothpastes and toothbrushes are now designed specifically for children to encourage good dental care.

Clothing

Parents need information and the opportunity to discuss practical aspects of clothing. Clothing should be relatively loose fitting, and appropriate to the weather and the temperature. Children's clothes should not have any cords or loose ties that could become caught around a limb or neck. Where possible clothes need to be practical and machine washable. Young children can get through quite a few clothing items in a day. Some strong washing powders and fabric conditioners may cause irritation to a baby's skin and need to be avoided where possible.

Psychological health

Crying

Crying is the only way that babies can attract attention or let us know that they want something. Small babies may cry because they are hungry, wet, tired, too hot or cold or just plain bored. Babies enjoy gentle touch, being spoken to and seeing people and objects. It is important to encourage parents to give this type of stimulation.

Babies also cry if they have wind, or

pain, and this can be distressing for parents and the child. There are many ways that babies can be helped with this, including medicines. Constant crying can be very frustrating for parents, and they may need support, information and help if they are becoming angry, losing sleep or saying that they cannot cope.

Toys

Unfortunately, not all toy manufacturers have safety in mind, and well intentioned parents and relatives may buy toys that are not appropriate for the child's age. Toys for babies should be soft, without eyes or noses that can be detached or swallowed, and have no sharp points. Most babies would prefer one large brightly coloured object like a mobile for them to look at and observe the movement. They may also enjoy a soft toy to touch and provide comfort. You may be required to remind parents about appropriate toys for children at different age stages.

Rivalry

Older children can feel left out or ignored when they have a new brother or sister. "Sibling rivalry" can be displayed by toddlers in many ways such as becoming withdrawn and introverted or having tantrums and outbursts of screaming. Parents need support to help them cope with this. It may include ensuring that they can give an adequate amount of attention to the older child and including them in the care of their younger brother or sister.

Child health surveillance

Although child development is monitored every day by parents and relatives, there is a common programme in the UK of developmental checks, often called child health surveillance. These are usually carried out in health centres and GP surgeries. Tables 2 and 3 contain details of

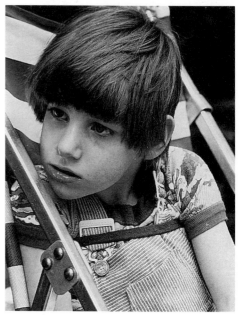

Every child's development is maintained in the UK by a system of regular checks.

child health reviews at different stages of the child's life.

Developmental assessments are offered by doctors and health visitors. Measuring the height, weight and head circumference, sight, hearing and developmental testing are examples of child health surveillance. You may be asked to assist in this activity in order to monitor progress and help to identify any problems.

Child health surveillance can never be 100 per cent accurate and may sometimes cause a false alarm or miss a problem. Occasionally a new problem may occur after the child has been assessed. Reporting and documenting your observations is therefore very important.

Record keeping

Although you will not be expected to interpret the results of tests, you may be required to record and document any results. Parent Held Records are common-

Table 2 – General questions at child health surveillance reviews
(Adapted from Camden & Islington Community Health Services Trust - Parent Held Records)

6- 8 weeks review
Do you feel well yourself?
Do you have any concerns about your baby's weight gain?
Does your baby watch your face and follow with their eyes?
Does your baby turn towards the light?
Does your baby smile at you?
Do you think your baby can hear you?
Is your baby startled by loud noises?
Are there any problems in looking after your baby?
Do you have any other worries?

3 months review
Has your baby had the first immunisation?
Does your baby laugh and gurgle?
Does your baby notice people/toys?
Does your baby watch their hands?
Does your baby quieten or smile to the sound of your voice even when you can't be seen?

Do you have any worries about your baby?

4 month review
Has your baby had the second immunisation?
Has your baby had any illnesses or accidents since the last check?
Have you been given advice about fluoride for your baby's teeth?
Do you have any worries about your baby?

6- 9 month review
Are you feeling well yourself?
Have you any worries about your child's health or development?
Do you have any worries about how your baby is feeding?
Are you happy your baby is gaining weight?
Is your baby sitting alone?
Does your baby babble (Ba-Ba, Da-da)?
Have you any worries about your baby's eyesight?
Have you noticed a squint (eyes not moving together?)
Do you think your baby can hear you?

ly used in the UK as well as professional records. Whatever type of records are used in your workplace, it is important that they are accurate and up to date. Records usually contain personal information through which you can identify the child, such as date of birth. This is important when immunisations and vaccines are being given by injection. They also record normal growth development and future health checks.

Parent Held Records are useful as they inform parents and can provide information on normal development and what to look out for. They also often contain information on safety at home and minor illness and ailments in childhood.

Records can be used as legal documents and should always be written clearly and as soon as possible after seeing the child or parent. Records should include the date, age of the child and measurement details.

A "centile" chart is commonly used to record and ensure that the weight, length and head circumference of babies and children are within a normal range. Centile charts look like a graph and are used as a guide to observing the actual and predicted growth of a child. This information should be shared with parents, but they should not be unduly worried if the chart does not appear to be perfect since there are many factors that can influence normal growth and development. You should receive instruction on how to complete the centile chart in use in your area.

In the clinic

Talking to parents as they arrive helps to create a welcoming atmosphere. It is helpful if you can show them around the clinic and give them an idea of the usual routine. If parents are required to wait, they will need reading material, play areas for children, health education leaflets and facilities to change nappies and wash babies.

These areas need to be clean, warm and safe from any dangers. Correct temperature is important as the body temperature of small babies can drop quickly, and naked babies may be at risk from draughts from open windows or doors.

You should ensure that all weighing equipment is thoroughly cleaned with a standard detergent before clinic sessions or if a child wets on the scales. A clean sheet of absorbent paper should be placed on the scales before each child is weighed. Weighing scales must be calibrated (checked) at each session to ensure that they give a correct reading.

Measuring growth
You may be required to help with the important task of measuring and recording the height, weight and head circumference of babies and children. A qualified member of staff will always be responsible for interpreting the measurements.

Weight
Regular weighing can be useful to identify

Table 3 – Child health surveillance 18-24 months

Are you feeling well yourself?
Have you any worries about your child's behaviour?
Are you happy your child is growing and hearing normally?
Does your child understand when you talk to him/her?
Do you have any worries about the way your child talks?
Are you happy that your child's eyesight is normal?
Do you think your child has a squint (eyes not moving together?)
Does your child walk normally?
Are you brushing your child's teeth every day?
Are your child's immunisations up-to-date?

Review at 3½ - 4 years
Have you any worries about your child's hearing, eyesight, speech, understanding of what you say, health, behaviour, potty training?
Can your child run, walk upstairs, stay dry by day?
Are all your child's immunisations up to date?

Review at 4½ - 5½ years
Have you any worries about your child?
Does your child wear glasses, hearing aid?
Has your child ever seen a specialist?
Does your child have any long-term health problems?
Does your child have any problems that may affect schooling?
Is your child clumsy?
Is your child dry day and night?
Does your child wheeze or have a night cough?
Do you have any worries about your child's health or behaviour?
Are your child's immunisations up to date including the pre-school booster?

those children who are not putting on weight, which is sometimes called "failure to thrive". It also reassures parents that their child is growing normally. Parents may be under-feeding or over-feeding their child. Some children may not be able to absorb certain milk feeds, which would need to be investigated.

It is important when weighing babies that you have been shown how to handle them confidently ensuring that their head is supported and limbs are positioned safely. Parents will become very nervous if they feel that their child is not safe in your hands.

Height and length

Children up to two years of age are usually measured lying down. A special mat with a foot and head board is used to accurately record their length. This is not a task that can easily be carried out alone. From the age of two years, standing height should be measured. Simple measuring sticks are not always accurate and "microtoise" or magnetic measuring devices should be used. The Child Growth Foundation provides details on the range of different devices.

Head circumference

Head circumference is usually measured at birth and again at six weeks of age. This is an indication of whether the child is growing proportionally, and if any further investigations need to be carried out. The tape measure is placed along the forehead and round the back of the head at the most prominent point. Although this is a simple procedure it should not be taken lightly. If you do not feel competent to undertake this activity after instruction always report back to a qualified member of staff.

Measuring vision

Measuring vision can range from very simple to very complicated tests, such as "visual acuity", which need to be carried out by

an orthoptist. You can, however look out for any abnormalities of the eyes, for example, sticky eyes, wandering eye movement, the inability of the child to follow the movement of a toy held in front of them, a dislike of sunlight (photophobia), or squinting. Always report any of these symptoms to a qualified member of staff.

Vision testing is important because it may identify children who are dyslexic, and poor vision may prevent a child from learning how to read and write. This can significantly affect their future.

On entering school and every three years, children are tested using special equipment. It is usual to test at a distance of three metres. If children can read, they are asked to read aloud single letters on a chart. Where children cannot read they are asked to match a shape to the one shown on the chart. You may be asked to help by holding a card over the child's eye so that each eye can be tested independently. A card with a pin hole may be used where children have difficulty with one or both eyes. Colour vision testing is usually carried out between the ages of 9 and 13.

Measuring hearing

The most common way of identifying hearing problems in children is when parents report that their child does not respond to their voice or loud noises. Hearing tests can identify children who may be deaf, or who have a condition known as "glue ear" which can lead to hearing loss. With all hearing testing it is important that the room is very quiet.

You should also have your hearing tested to ensure that you can test others.

A distraction test is usually carried out at six to eight months. You may be required to be the "tester" whilst a qualified member of staff will be the distracter.

School age children are tested using an audiometer machine. The child wears a set of headphones and indicates to the tester when they can or cannot hear a noise played to them.

Immunisations

Immunisation involves injecting the child with a safe dose of a virus in order to build up their defences (immunity) to disease. The immune system in the body then recognises the virus if exposed to it in the future and is usually able to destroy it. The common vaccines given to children in the UK are diphtheria, whooping cough, tetanus, polio, measles, mumps and rubella. In the UK immunisation programmes can start in the first six weeks of a child's life.

BCG, a vaccine used to protect children from tuberculosis, can be given to babies almost immediately after birth, but is more commonly given only to babies at high risk of contracting tuberculosis at the age of two weeks to six weeks.

You may be required to hold children securely and safely whilst they are being injected, as some parents do not like to do this. Wrapping a child in a clean blanket and exposing the arm or leg for injection is one of the safest ways of preventing the child from wriggling and moving.

Some children may have a mild reaction to immunisation soon after injection. They may develop a temperature and become irritable and cry. If parents are not informed of these side effects it can cause unnecessary anxiety and worry. You may need to repeat information given to parents about removing clothing to reduce temperature and giving frequent cooled drinks. Some health professionals will also advise parents to administer specific medicines. Health education leaflets describing vaccines and immunisation should be accessible in each place of immunisation. Remember that you may need to get copies of these in languages other than English.

Teenagers

The teenage years are a confusing time for many young people as so many physical, emotional and social changes are taking place. Young people become more interested in their own bodies and become sexually mature. Girls begin to develop breasts and start to have periods while boys develop muscular changes and deeper voices. Both girls and boys start to take a sexual interest in others around them.

Young people need the opportunity to confide in others and to talk about these changes and the way that they feel. Many teenagers do not feel that they can share their thoughts with parents and may turn to school nurses or teachers.

There are specific plans set out by the Government for providing health education to school age children. It is important however, to be aware of the main risks in this age group. These include motor vehicle and bicycle accidents, introduction to and experimentation with drugs and alcohol, and sexual activity without protection from pregnancy or sexually transmitted diseases such as HIV. Specially designed information leaflets are available on all these subjects from local health education departments.

A number of other social service, teaching and voluntary workers, such as social workers and playleaders are also able to contribute to ensuring good child health. They are in a position to see children in familiar surroundings and may detect problems of delayed development. Close working with other child care agencies is essential for promoting healthy childhood.

Points to remember

1. A knowledge of the way in which children grow and develop is important to understand how things may go wrong or why illness may occur in later life.

2. It is also important that the health and wellbeing of parents are safeguarded by reinforcing information and providing support.

3. Good physical and emotional health requires good nutrition, appropriate clothing, meeting emotional needs and having the opportunity to participate in the normal activities of life.

4. Child development is monitored every day by parents and relatives and there is a programme of developmental checks in the UK, often called child health surveillance.

5. You may be asked to assist in child health surveillance activity, such as weighing, measuring and participating in vision and hearing testing of children.

6. An important factor in preventing disease is childhood immunisation.

7. Children reaching adulthood also need to have their health needs considered and to receive advice about healthy lifestyles.

8. Close working with other child care agencies, such as social workers and teachers is essential for promoting healthy childhood.

Resources
Health Education Authority
Hamilton House
Mabledon Place
London WC1 H9TX
071-383-3833

Further reading
Morton J, McFarlane A (1991) *Child Health and Surveillance*. Blackwell Scientific, London.
Hall D (1992) *Health for all children*. Oxford University Press, Oxford.

NVQ Levels 2 & 3 Core Units
O Promote equality for all individuals.
U4 Contribute to the health, safety and security of individuals and their environment.
U5 Obtain, transmit and store information relating to the delivery of a care service.

Level 3 Core Units
Z4 Promote communication with clients where there are communication difficulties.
Y2 Enable clients to make use of available services and information.

CHAPTER 9

Living with a physical disability

Marion Judd and Veronica Beasley

• Quality of life and independence • Identifying problem areas • Problems around the home • Living alone • Dressing and hygiene • Walking aids and footwear • Your vital link

Most people take their ability to perform ordinary activities of daily living for granted. People who are "physically able", automatically walk where and when they please. They are able to wash, dress and feed themselves and take part in social and recreational activities. To be "physically disabled" means that ordinary everyday tasks and activities may be difficult or even impossible.

Physical disability can be acquired at any time of life. Some people are born with disabilities caused by conditions such as cerebral palsy or spina bifida. Others become disabled as a result of accidents and adults of all ages may become disabled as a result of diseases such as multiple sclerosis or motor neurone disease.

Disability can have a profound effect on a person's quality of life. They may no longer be able to do all those automatic everyday activities and thus disability can affect their independence, choice and lifestyle.

It is very important that people are offered the right help to enable them to enjoy the best quality of life and to remain active, independent and safe in their own home. Keeping as fit and as mobile as possible helps to reduce the level of disability, and disabled people have the right to professional help to enable them do this.

You may be the person who spends the most time with the client. Getting to know them better and observing how they perform activities of daily living will enable you to identify particular problems. You may ask questions like this:

- "Is that difficult?"
- "What is the problem, is it your shoulders/wrists/hands/hips?"
- "Is it painful?"
- "That looks a struggle!"
- "Can you get to the toilet in time?"
- "Would you like to be able to do it?"

These questions may encourage the client to talk about their problems, or pave the way for reporting problems to a qualified member of staff or suggesting that referral to an occupational therapist (OT) or physiotherapist is needed.

Around the home

To illustrate some of the problems a client may have, we will go on a tour of their home. The following are suggestions for the sorts of things you may need to look out for, which can help a client to remain independent and safe at home.

The garden gate

One of the first things to consider is access to a person's home. If there is a garden gate, can the client operate the latch? Is it too large, too small, too heavy, spring loaded, or does it swing in the wrong direction?

The path to the front door

Non-slip, even floor surfaces and pavements are very important for people who may have difficulty walking. Steps and edges of paths may need to be clearly visible and wide enough for clients with a stick, frame, trolley or wheelchair. Although many people have handrails to help them, these may have been fixed on the wrong side for the client, or they may need rails on two sides.

The front door

If a client cannot hear the doorbell, it is possible for a flashing light to be installed to replace the bell. A spyhole, positioned so that the client can use it, can add to safety and prevent unwanted callers from entering the home. Alternatively, an entry-phone, sited in a convenient place in the home, may be easier for people who cannot reach the door quickly.

Clients with a visual difficulty may not be able to see the door lock or be able to hold a key. Special key holders are available for clients with a weak grip. Lever type door handles are much easier to operate than knobs. Difficult steps can sometimes be removed and retractable ones or a ramp can be fitted.

A letter box cage fixed to the door can save the client from bending to pick up mail; however it may prevent the door from being opened wide enough to allow the client to get through the door in a passage or entrance hall. A pick up stick ("helping hand" – Fig 1) could be used instead to enable a client who is unable to bend, to pick up mail and other objects from the floor.

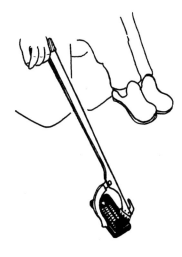

Fig 1. "Helping hand" or pick-up stick.

Entrance hall/passageway

Mats and rugs: Loose mats anywhere can be hazardous, particularly frayed ones. If possible, it is better not to have any. However, a client may not want them removed, in which case they need to be trimmed if frayed, and secured with either tacks or double-sided sticky carpet tape. Mats on wood, tiled or linoleum floors can be secured by placing non-slip strips under them. Door mat recesses can be a hazard if the mat does not fit the recess or where the mat has worn down.

Lighting: Well lit hallways and stairs are particularly important to avoid the danger of tripping and falling. Clients may agree to move furniture or obstacles to ensure that they can manoeuvre in small spaces, particularly if they are using sticks, frames or trolleys.

In the kitchen

Light switches and plugs
Large rocker-type electric switches, and special sockets and plugs are available where a client's reach or hand function is limited. These need to be sited at a suitable level for the client. Plugs can be fitted with special handles to assist clients with weak, painful or deformed hands (Fig 2).

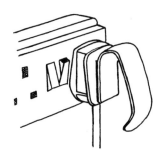

Fig 2. Plug with special handle.

Taps
For clients with limited hand function, equipment is available to convert taps to lever controls which the client can operate. These can be obtained for clients who are unable to stand at the sink or while performing other kitchen tasks.

Ovens
If a client cannot bend or reach into a conventional oven, ovens can be raised on plinths, or an alternative worktop oven or microwave oven may be supplied. Clients who are unable to stand without support may benefit from a "perching stool" (Fig 3). This will enable them to have both hands free to prepare food and drinks.

Windows
Opening or closing windows across a worktop can be difficult for able-bodied

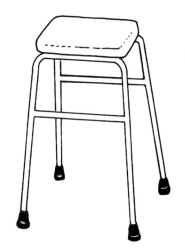

Fig 3 Perching stool.

people and impossible for people with a disability. Equipment such as remote controlled winding gear or alternatively a plastic air vent can be inserted into the window.

Kitchen activities
Most clients are keen to be as active as possible around the kitchen. There are many pieces of equipment available which can assist independence. These include:
• long-handled dustpan and brush
• long-handled milk bottle holders
• easy to operate tin openers
• wire baskets which fit in saucepans to save lifting heavy pans
• one-handed whisks
• large-handled and insulated mugs
• specially designed plates and bowls
• large-handled cutlery
• kettle tippers (Fig 4)
• lightweight utensils.

In the living room

Armchairs and settees are often low, squashy and difficult to get out of for a disabled client. Armrests help, but if the seat is low the client may resort to sitting on a dining-room type chair. In most cases, chairs can be raised, either by fitting leg extenders or a platform to go under the chair. If the chair is very soft, plywood can be cut to size and placed under the seat cushion. It is important that the client's feet touch the ground, or are placed on an easily moved footrest. Furniture may also need re-positioning to improve access and mobility and increase independence.

For some clients, television, radio and telephones may be the only contact with other people for long periods of time, so they need to be easily accessible. Telephones with large, push button numbers can be made available if a client has visual problems. Loudspeakers and "Hearing Loop" systems can also be made available. Your district OT should be able to advise.

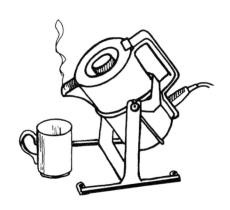

Fig 4 Kettle tipper.

Living alone

A few clients may use their dependence on others to gain social contacts as they live alone and are isolated. These clients may become anxious at any encouragement towards being more independent. They will need reassurance that care will not be withdrawn if they become able to take a more active part in their activities of daily living.

In the bedroom

Beds

Some clients find getting in and out of bed so difficult that they resort to sleeping in a chair; this can cause swelling of the legs and feet which may then affect their mobility and general health. An old bed with a squashy mattress can make the movement from sitting to standing more difficult. Sometimes a board under the mattress, to provide a firm support from which to rise, makes it easier for the client to get up or transfer to a wheelchair.

The physiotherapist or occupational therapist can advise and teach clients how to sit up in bed, get out of bed and how to transfer from beds to chairs. "Rope ladders" and "monkey poles" are types of equipment that the client can use to assist themselves in some circumstances. (See also chapter 16, Lifting and handling.)

Commodes

If a commode is placed by the bed, this can remove the worry of "having an accident". A night-light may be a further comfort, especially if the client finds it difficult to locate the bedside switch when awaking from sleep.

Dressing and undressing

Dressing and undressing can be a fiddly process at the best of times. Appropriate fastenings on clothes can help the client to preserve their dignity and remain independent. Additionally, equipment for pulling on socks and stockings can be made available where people cannot bend or stretch.

Bathroom and toilet

Getting on and off the toilet safely, being able to wash at the hand basin and getting into and out of the bath are the main areas of concern for the person with a disability. An enormous range of additional equipment and permanent adaptations can be made available.

Toilets

Where the bathroom and toilet are separate, assisting a disabled client into a narrow toilet can be awkward or dangerous, especially if the client uses a walking frame or a wheelchair. Transferring onto a chair with wheels and a commode hole in the seat may help. This can then be pushed back over the toilet pan with the client already on board.

Baths, showers and hand basins

Many types of bath boards, seats and hand rails (and hoists) can be obtained according to the client's and carer's needs.

Walking aids

You may be the first person to observe that a client is unsteady on their feet or unsafe to walk alone, and may be helped by using a walking aid. The most commonly used walking aids are walking sticks and walking frames. Both come in a variety of shapes and sizes to cater for different clients' needs. All sticks and frames should have rubber feet (ferrules) to prevent the walking aid from slipping when the client leans on it.

Each individual person should be assessed by a physiotherapist or OT and provided with their own safe walking aid. They should be measured to ensure that they are the correct height and that the grip is comfortable for the client's hand.

Walking frames

Clients who are unsteady on their feet but able to walk safely with extra support, may find it easier and safer to use a walking frame. Walking frames are made of metal. Most frames are adjustable in height and come in a variety of widths to suit the client and the client's home. Folding frames are available for clients who go out in a car.

Frames with special handgrips are available to suit individual needs; for example clients with rheumatoid arthritis may need grips specially moulded for their hands. Frame bags are also available so that clients can carry their belongings with them.

The client's technique with the frame is important for their safety. You can help by encouraging them to move exactly as instructed by the OT when walking or rising from a chair.

Frames that are too wide for doorways and passages are no use at all.

Walking sticks

Wooden walking sticks are best for most people. They last a lifetime without deteriorating, can be easily cut to the right height, can hook securely over an arm to leave the client's hands free, and have a comfortable grip for most people. Metal, adjustable sticks with special handgrips are available. Over time, however, the holes in a metal stick tend to wear, making the stick noisy to use.

Footwear

Well fitting shoes and slippers make walking easier and safer for most people. Safe, non-slip footwear can help to prevent falls, and specialised footwear and appliances for extra foot and ankle support may be needed. Physiotherapists and podiatrists are a source of expert advice on safe and practical footwear.

Your vital link

The care assistant provides a vital link between the client and qualified members of staff. Addressing practical and safety problems can mean the difference between a client being able to live at home in the community or going into residential care. Being observant, listening to the client and clearly reporting any findings to a qualified member of staff so that appropriate referrals can be made, are essential. Professional advice is available from physiotherapists and occupational therapists for both small aids and equipment and where extensive alterations may be needed in the home. It is important to recognise however that some people, for a variety of reasons, may not want to have aids, adaptations or changes in their home, and their feelings must always be respected.

Points to remember

1. To be "physically disabled" means that ordinary everyday tasks and activities are difficult or even impossible.
2. Physical disability can be acquired at any time of life. Some people are born with disabilities, others become disabled as a result of accidents and adults of all ages may become disabled as a result of disease.
3. It is very important that people are offered the right help, keep as fit and mobile as possible and are referred to occupational therapists and physiotherapists to enable them to remain active, independent and safe in their own home.
4. The care assistant's vital contribution is to be observant, listening to the client and clearly reporting any findings to a qualified member of staff so that appropriate referrals can be made.
5. There is a wide range of small aids and equipment as well as major home adapta-

tions for every room in the home, that can be used to promote independence. The OT can advise.
6. Sticks and frames should be measured for each client and kept in good repair.
7. Well fitting, non-slip shoes are essential to promote mobility and to prevent tripping and falls.

NVQ Level 2 &3 Core Units
O Promote equality for all individuals.
U4 Contribute to the health, safety and security of individuals and their environment.
U5 Obtain, transmit and store information relating to the delivery of a care service.

Level 2 Core Units
W2 Contribute to the ongoing support of clients and others significant to them.
W3 Support clients in transition due to their care requirements.

Level 3 Core Units
Z4 Promote communication with clients where there are communication difficulties.
Y2 Enable clients to make use of available services and information.

Level 2 Direct Care
Z6 Enable clients to maintain and improve their mobility.
Z7 Contribute to the movement and treatment of clients to maximise their physical comfort.
Z9 Enable clients to maintain their personal hygiene and appearance.
Z10 Enable clients to eat and drink.
Z11 Enable clients to access and use toilet facilities.
Z19 Enable clients to achieve physical comfort.

Level 2 Domiciliary Support
Z7 Contribute to the movement and treatment of clients to maximise their physical comfort.
W8 Enable clients to maintain contacts in potentially islolating situations.
U1 Contribute to the maintenance and management of domestic and personal resources.

CHAPTER 10

Caring for people with learning disabilities

Hilary Brown

• Who are "people with learning disabilities" and what are their needs? • The legacy of institutional care • Communication and frustration • Providing physical or intimate care • Helping people with daily household tasks • Helping people to learn new skills

The wide range of people who are described by this label means that, for a care assistant, the work can vary enormously. Many people with learning disabilities live almost independently with a little help from a paid worker, perhaps in finding a job or paying the bills, while others will depend on their families or on carers within residential settings for help with almost all their daily needs. Some people will be able to make choices and state their preferences while others may need support in acting in their best interests.

Who are people with learning disabilities?

Until recently people with learning disabilities were referred to as mentally handicapped, but the change of term to "learning disability" is more respectful and makes clearer the difficulties which people have. It conveys an expectation that, with the right kind of help, people can learn and develop, also it avoids confusion with people who have "mental illness" or

are suffering from emotional distress. In short, people with learning disabilities are neither "mad", "bad" nor "sad", just people who are likely to find learning more difficult than other people and to need specific help in the course of their everyday lives.

Learning disabilities are difficulties acquired before, at, or soon after birth, so that they affect the whole of a person's development. Common causes are chromosomal abnormalities at or around conception, of which the most common is Down's syndrome; the results of a virus or illness the mother has during pregnancy as in rubella; or brain damage caused by trauma during birth which sometimes causes cerebral palsy with or without learning disabilities.

Sometimes the cause of a person's disabilities cannot be accurately pinpointed, and sometimes it will only be noticed gradually as the mother or father become anxious that their daughter or son is not reaching the usual milestones. If there is a known cause of the person's difficulties you may want to find out more about it, not so you can pigeon-hole them, but so that you can be alert to any additional difficulties they may have. For example people with Down's Syndrome may have visual or hearing problems, and young women with spina bifida may start their periods unusually early. Your local library should be able to help you find relevant information.

Be clear about your role

The nature of your role as a care assistant will need to be discussed very fully with all the parties involved so that you and they are clear about what you are there to do. You will need to clarify how much of your time is to be spent supporting the person's relative or carer rather than working with the person with a learning disability her or himself.

Being clear at the beginning is important. Otherwise you might find that you drift into helping and talking to the person's carer, especially if you find the person with a learning disability difficult, unpredictable, or not easy to communicate with. You should have a clear plan or contract about why you are there and what sort of help you are supposed to give.

We need to consider some background issues to help you put the work you are doing with individuals into some sort of context. It is important to look at what kind of services people with learning disabilities received in the past and at the principles on which services are now designed.

The old hospitals

On the edge of most towns and cities you will still find old fashioned "subnormality" hospitals where all the people with learning disabilities from a particular neighbourhood used to live. Often they were behind walls and offered care in large dormitories and villas where all the housework would be done for people and few if any of the rhythms of everyday life would apply.

On the positive side many of the hospitals had nice grounds and caring staff, but the disadvantages tended to outweigh the good points. People had no privacy, if they wanted a cup of tea they could not just go and get one, they had meals cooked in a central kitchen, often served lukewarm and without choices or the opportunity to shop and cook for your favourite dishes. You couldn't turn the fire up if you were cold or stay up if you fancied watching a late film on TV.

People would have few opportunities to use local facilities. Mostly they were just bored. One researcher (Oswin 1971) called her book about life in hospitals at the weekend (when many staff had time off) *The empty hours*, and the image which many visitors had was of people sitting around the edge of the room rocking or picking at their clothes, desperately trying to find something to do with their time until the next meal or bathtime would relieve the waiting. Parents and family members often had to travel long distances or make expensive journeys; inevitably sometimes people lost touch.

New challenges

It is useful to go over this history for several reasons. Firstly, because it helps you to see why newer services place such an emphasis on being just like other houses and not marking people with learning disabilities out or removing them from their local communities and networks.

Secondly, it is important to remember that many people who receive help in group homes and hostels are people who have lived in such hospitals. They may experience difficulties in doing ordinary things not because of their learning disability but because they have never had the

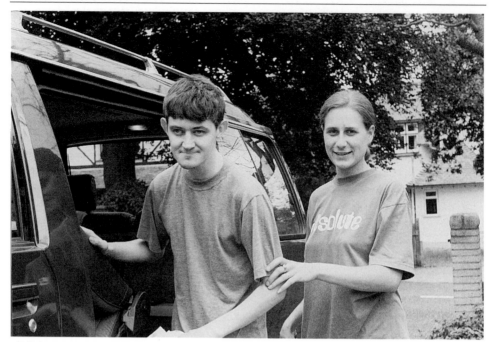

Off for a swim: your encouragement and support will make it possible for people with learning disabilities to join in a whole range of activities in the community.

chance to try things out. They may have developed mannerisms or phrases which were appropriate on the ward but are not useful in their new home. They may have withdrawn into a private world.

Moving will be a major change in their way of life and they will need to learn new skills and face up to new challenges. Living in a busy street may be daunting if you are not used to it; so will learning to do the weekly shop in a supermarket. Often moving out allows people who used to live at home before they were placed in hospital (often when their parents or family members could no longer manage due to illness or getting older) to take up again where they left off: for others these things are completely new.

Research suggests that when people first move out there is a very rapid growth in their skills, but that after a while progress towards independence levels off unless a really consistent effort is made to develop

new opportunities and help people to make the most of them.

That is where you come in: it isn't the move which will change things for people with learning disabilities – you can be lonely and sit around all day in your local neighbourhood – it is the encouragement and support you can give which makes it possible for people to join in a whole range of activities and meet people. Sometimes your job will be to help with practical tasks, sometimes to challenge prejudice or pity by showing other members of the public that people with learning disabilities are individuals who are worthy of respect.

Ordinary lives

Knowing about the history of services also helps to make sense of the language you will hear from staff: it will help you to understand why people wanted to change stigmatising terms like mentally subnormal, cripple, and stop lumping people together as "the mentally handicapped". It also provides a background to the idea of "normalisation", because it is partly in response to such services that policies changed so drastically that now the goal is to make it possible for people with learning disabilities to live more "ordinary" lives and take up their place in their local communities.

There are lots of different versions of "normalisation", some of which make more sense than others, but basically they argue that people with learning disabilities have the right to lead as ordinary a life as possible and that it is the job of staff to make that possible. Normalisation doesn't mean just standing back and not interfering: it means finding ways of helping which make new things possible.It doesn't mean pretending that the person doesn't have a handicap but working to minimise the effect of any impairment on their daily lives. It means encouraging people to make their own choices but not allowing people to take unjustified risks or leaving them open to abuse.

Balancing act

It is this balancing act which you have to learn: for one person it might mean constructing a communication board so they can ask for their choice of drink when they want one; for another it might mean opening up a bank account and helping them to manage their money. For someone else it might mean a weekly trip to the pub or to a football match, or arranging a lift to church.

One framework which might help you to decide priorities is John O' Brien's five accomplishments (O'Brien 1986). He established that the goal for everyone is to help them belong, and suggested that to do that you have to be present in the community and in ordinary places like swimming pools, doctors' surgeries, shops and offices, not in segregated places like day centres or special hydrotherapy pools, or in hostels where the doctor comes to you, rather than you going to her.

You have to be given choices and be allowed to develop tastes and preferences (such as how long you like your boiled eggs cooked and whether you take one or two sugars in your tea). Also you have to be helped to develop your own confidence and competence by being taught new skills in a professional and consistent way, not just left to learn by trial and error.

Respect

Throughout, you need to make sure that the person is treated with respect, not talked down to, or in front of. People with learning disabilities are often treated as if they have no status, and if those supporting them do not challenge this, members of the public will not get the message. This sounds easy but it may not always be so. Sometimes people with learning disabilities are difficult to be with; they may do things which you disapprove of, or which you find annoying. You will have to help them in ways that other adults are not helped, and yet the skill is in helping them without making it obvious and in speaking about them with understanding rather than blame.

Because the group of people labelled as having learning disabilities varies so much, there is no way a chapter like this can tell you exactly how to work with each individual, but it can tell you what to look out for. Most services will draw up an individual plan to guide the work with each person, and you can ask to be included in that process by giving your ideas. You may also be asked to work towards some of the goals which have been identified on the person's plan, such as teaching them a particular skill, or you may be asked to work in an agreed way, such as responding to difficult behaviour in the same way as other staff so that the person gets a consistent response.

Communication ...and frustration

Communication is at the core of caring for people and is bound to be an issue for most people: that means both being able to listen to and understand what the person is saying to you, and being able to let them know what you are doing and what the plans are for your time together.

Many people with learning disabilities manage speech and language with no problems, but for others there are major barriers to making themselves understood. Many people with learning disabilities *are* able to make their views clear but are handicapped by the fact that other people won't listen to them or act on what they say. If people do find it difficult to say what they want, this might be because of physical problems with their speech, or it might reflect the fact that they have fewer words at their disposal.

You also need to check out how much individuals understand – what they can say and what they understand may be two different things. Sometimes people with learning disabilities rely on single words in a sentence, so that if you say "we are not going shopping tomorrow" they only respond to the word "shopping" and get very confused at the lack of action on your part! Different tenses, for example "went" or "will go" might be difficult, as well as other words which describe time, for example, before, after or tomorrow. Also negatives such as "we didn't get the video" can be too complicated for some people.

Also, many people have additional problems such as hearing impairment and visual handicaps: you should always be alert

Making a plan for each individual

• Be clear about how you are going to spend your time with the person you are helping.

• Try to balance the needs of the person with learning disabilities and her or his carer: don't spend all your time with the carer.

• Find out how much the person understands and how they express themselves.

• Be alert to the possibility that the person may have additional problems such as a hearing impairment or difficulty in seeing

• Don't blame the person for any difficult behaviour but work out a consistent way of managing it.

• Remember that the behaviour may be the person's best effort at communicating with you or making things happen around them; it could be the person's way of getting a bit of peace, or of asking for something, or simply of passing time if they are bored or can't get involved in more interesting activities.

• Become a bit of a detective and try to work out what they need in the situation, and help them to get what they need without hurting themselves or others if you can.

• Remember to take the person's own culture and routines into account; you must adjust to them, not the other way around.

• If other professionals are involved, ask them how you should approach different situations with the person you are helping.

and if the person acts in a way you did not expect, try to work out why. Perhaps they usually rely on gestures or on watching others to help them make sense of what is happening: people may appear to have more language skills because they are good at seeing what staff or carers are going to do next or because they know the routine of the place.

Many people with learning disabilities use alternative forms of communication either to augment or replace speech. The most common alternatives are signing and the use of picture or symbol boards to which they can point. You will need to become proficient in using these kinds of communication. Sometimes people use their eyes, or gestures to indicate yes or no, and you will need to present them with appropriate options so they can tell you what they want through a series of questions.

Attention seeking?

Because people with learning disabilities sometimes have problems in understanding what is going on around them and also have difficulty in telling others what they want, they may fall back on behaviours which are difficult for others to deal with. For example they may shout or become aggressive or hurt themselves by banging their head or biting the back of their hand. Each of these behaviours is likely to be saying something.

The usual response from staff is that the person is "attention seeking", but that may not be the answer. It may be that they are finding your presence too difficult to deal with, that the task in hand is too complex, that they are hungry or thirsty or in pain. A psychologist may have written up a programme telling you how to respond to particular behaviours, and will base this on their understanding of the causes of the person's difficult behaviour. They may well want ideas from you about what happens before or after the behaviour which can give you clues as to what the person needs.

Physical or intimate care

People who need physical care will need you to help in a down to earth manner, without getting embarrassed or drawing attention to their bodies in an unpleasant way. You need to find a balance between being very "professional" and distant, which could seem as if you are looking down at them, and being over-familiar.

Try to take your cue from them about how to behave: ask them to tell you if you have done something in the way they like it to be done, and above all remember how important it is to you to be comfortable, so you can take the same care as you would want taken yourself. If you are bathing the person, help to make this a pleasant rather than just a hygienic experience, dry them carefully to make sure that they do not get sore, and help them to dress in clothes they like and feel comfortable in. There is nothing worse than having your bra strap crossed or your shirt bunched up all day!

The daily round

In our lives we tend to be always busy, and it is tempting to get chores over and done with as quickly as possible. But remember, for people with learning disabilities it is more likely that they don't have *enough* interesting things to do.

The golden rule is always to do things *with* them rather than *for* them. Even if they can only do a little part of the job it is more satisfying for you to do it together than for them to be left alone while you get on with it for convenience's sake. Perhaps if you are peeling potatoes for lunch, they can wash the potatoes and you can peel them, or if you are making sandwiches they can butter the bread and you can make the fillings. Remember you aren't doing anyone any favours if you "use up" all the things the person could have done for themselves, unless of course you have something more exciting than housework planned for the day!

Doing specific jobs, such as budgeting with or on behalf of the person if they can't manage

It may be that you are there to give some very specific help such as helping the person to manage their money or do their shopping. If so, make sure that you consult them and only step in with the parts of the task they need help with. For example if the reason the person needs help with shopping is because they use a wheelchair and have difficulty lifting things off the top shelf and putting items into the trolley, you do not need to help them choose what they are going to eat.

Helping people to learn new skills they can then use independently

Because of their impairments people with learning disabilities are likely to find it more difficult to learn just by "taking things in", and will need those around them to think through the best way of doing things in order to teach a particular skill the same way each time.

Have you ever been half way through making pastry with flour all over your hands and then found that you have forgotten to switch the oven on? You end up getting flour all over the oven switches and/or putting the pastry in a cold oven. If you are helping someone with a learning disability to learn a new skill, you need to think it through for them until they get the hang of it, doing any bits which they can't manage and making sure you have got everything ready in advance. That way they get the sense of having succeeded: you help them through any "sticky bits" until they are secure in what they have

learned, and then step by step you help them to do the whole job.

Helping people to join in by going out with them to use shops or other facilities or to take part in leisure and sporting activities

Choosing activities and networks for people to join in is an important aspect of the caring role. You need to go to places where you meet the same people each time and where conversation is easy. Sometimes the art is in using your own contacts and approaching individuals in the community to ask if they will act as a "bridge".

For example you might say to someone, "David is a Baptist and I wondered if you might introduce him at your church: he'd love to go again as he hasn't been able to go since his mother died". Sometimes such a request is met with hostility, but usually this just masks a fear of embarrassment and/or a feeling that they may not know how to help.

Giving more detailed information will often be enough. For example you could explain that David enjoys singing but probably wouldn't want to stay in church for the sermon, so asking if he could help to make the refreshments would be good; or if the person needed more help you could make sure that a member of staff would accompany him, thereby reassuring your friend at the church that they would not need to disrupt their own routine. Often it is practical things like getting a lift, or finding a way for somebody to be involved, like taking the collection or collecting the hymn books, which can make all the difference.

Spending time with the person, listening to them and responding to their feelings and wishes

If someone finds it difficult to express themselves it may take you longer to get to know them, and can be frustrating for you in conversation as well as for them. While you are with them however, you should make a point of spending some time to concentrate on what they are trying to tell you so that you take an interest in, and build up your understanding of, what their life feels like.

Don't always expect them to be cheerful, or saintly. Also don't always back off difficult issues. Sometimes people with learning disabilities have to bite back feeling envious of their brothers and sisters, or feeling lonely.

Instead of saying "how lovely" when you are looking at family wedding photos, you might help the person say how they feel about relationships. Sometimes people with learning disabilities are well aware that they are treated differently from other people: they may wish for a partner and be sad that they are not married; they may want children but see that it is unlikely; they may be gay and feel isolated because no one acknowledges their sexuality.

People with learning disabilities are sometimes abused, physically or sexually, usually by someone they know who may be in a position of trust or authority, so be alert to what is being said and if they do disclose abuse do report it further so that it can be looked into. If someone has abused one person with a learning disability they may go on to hurt others: they need to be stopped.

Relieving their carer for a while so that they are able to go out or spend time on their own

Part of your job may be to relieve the carer who usually has responsibility for looking after the person. In this case you must consider and balance their needs as well as the needs of the person they care for. It may be that if you can be clear you can come up with some imaginative ways of being together.

For example one care assistant was asked to "babysit" for a man with learning disabilities every Thursday night and his mother, for whom this was her only night off, had resisted suggestions that Michael could also have an outing on the same evening. It became clear that her reasons were well founded: she knew that if Michael was going out as well, she would have to spend the time she had for getting ready herself helping him to get ready, and also she did not want to lose her evening to herself if he was unwell or if the club he was going to was cancelled.

When Mary the care assistant understood these objections, she was able to make a plan which included her helping Michael to get ready, and also which gave Michael's mother a guarantee that if Michael's activity was cancelled she would still come to sit with him.

Once Michael's mother had been assured that her own needs would be respected, she was happy for Michael to be going out. Mary and Michael have meanwhile been going to a local Irish club where they both enjoy the music and the atmosphere.

Mary has also found a way to help with the laundry. She puts a load of washing on while she helps Michael get ready and puts it into the tumble dryer before they go out, folding it after she has put Michael to bed when they get back. In this case recognising the carer's need first made it possible to do something more interesting for Michael without putting an extra burden on his mother.

Supporting the person's carer

Sometimes caring can get on top of people: it is very hard physical work as well as being emotionally stressful. Carers are often worried about the future, their own aches and pains signal to them that they will not always be able to care for their relative and they may also need advice as the needs of their relative change.

It is inevitable that sometimes carers will feel hard done by and may need a shoulder to cry on or someone to moan at. You may be able to help by feeding back your understanding of their needs to the care manager, and alerting them if you think that more help or specific guidance is needed.

Conclusion

Balancing people's needs and seeing a way forward is at the heart of caring for people with learning disabilities. It takes a lot of commitment and a very clear sense that individuals have a right to help and understanding from their local community, and that carers have a right to support in the work they do. Standing up for people doesn't mean getting into fights on their behalf, but it does mean calmly challenging prejudice and refusing to see people with learning disabilities treated as second class citizens.

Points to remember

1. Have a plan of how you are going to use your time with the person.
2. Try to do things in the same way each time so that the person learns that there is a pattern.
3. Be diplomatic when you are out and about with the person you are helping. Speak out for their rights, challenge people who say that they shouldn't be "seen" or shouldn't use the pub or the library, tell them that people with learning disabilities have the same rights as other citizens.
4. Don't just stand back, make positive plans with, and for, the person you are caring for.
5. Spend a certain amount of time really concentrating on the person, what they want and how they feel. Learn how they communicate and what their interests are.
6. Take advice from others on how to help someone who has difficult behaviours: remember it's not their fault and they aren't doing it deliberately, or aiming it at you personally.
7. Be encouraging to the person and their family members. Remember life can be difficult for everyone sometimes.
8. Don't expect people with learning disabilities to be "jolly" all the time: they too get depressed and sad and have to deal with feeling envious, or being bereaved. Ordinary feelings are a part of ordinary life.

Further reading
A Practical Guide to Working with People with Learning Disabilities. Edited by Hilary Brown and Sue Benson. Hawker Publications, London.
Oswin M (1971) *The empty hours: A study of the weekend life of handicapped children in institutions* Allen Lane, London.
O'Brien J (1986) A guide to personal futures planning, *The activities catalogue: a community programming guide for youth and adults with severe disabilities.* Bellamy and Wilcox (editors) Paul Brookes, New York.
Bringing People Back Home – training videos available from Pavilion Publishing, Brighton.

NVQ Levels 2 & 3 Core Units
O Promote equality for all individuals.
U4 Contribute to the health, safety and security of individuals and their environment.
U5 Obtain, transmit and store information relating to the delivery of a care service.

Level 2 Core Unit
W2 Contribute to the ongoing support of clients and others significant to them.

Level 3 Core Units
Z4 Promote communication with clients where there are communication difficulties.
Z8 Support clients when they are distressed.
Y2 Enable clients to make use of available services and information.

Level 2 Direct Care
Z6 Enable clients to maintain and improve their mobility.

Level 2 Domiciliary Support
Y1 Enable clients to manage their domestic and personal resources.
W8 Enable clients to maintain contacts in potentially isolating situations.

CHAPTER 11

A healthy old age

Eric Midwinter

• Taking a broad view • Active older people in the community • Statistics
• Old does not mean ill • Encouraging independence and choice

Being old is normal. Nearly 12 million people in the United Kingdom are over 60 years of age; almost a fifth of the population. Contrary to popular belief, the number living in care is very small. About 330,000 older people (less than three per cent of those over 60) live in residential homes, nursing homes, sheltered housing and so on. The vast majority live at home.

Being very old as opposed to old is not so exceptional either. Nearly four million people are over 75, and there are 180,000 over the age of 90. You will probably find that you provide care for more older women than older men. This reflects what happens in society at large where women gradually grow in numbers compared to men as they get older.

We are living in an "old" society. The chief reason why the proportion of older people has risen dramatically, is because the proportion of younger people has dropped dramatically. A hundred years ago near enough to two-fifths of the population was under 14; that has halved to one fifth. It is unlikely to change significantly.

Old does not mean ill

Although many people are in your care for reasons of ill health, it is worth recalling that "old" does not mean "ill" . By the very token of increased survival into older age, it follows that a decline in health should not automatically be associated with an increase in years.

Consider the following statements, based on an over-75 yardstick. These are, of course, national figures, for all over 75s. Let us assume a sample group of 100 people over 75 years of age.

This 100 were asked had they suffered any "restricted activity" during the previous fortnight, any time they had been inhibited from getting about in the ordinary way. Seventy five of them had not been so restricted. Asked if they were housebound or bedfast, 90 of them said they weren't. Asked if they were able to climb the stairs without assistance, 86 said they could do that in reasonable comfort.

You see, if you put the figures the other way round, they do look a little sunnier and more optimistic. Of course, it is bad enough that 25 out of every 100 people over 75 have been limited in activity during the last two weeks. But it's not a complete tale of woe.

It is just too risky to assume that everyone over-75 is automatically declining in health and capability at some alarming rate. Take dementia. The popular view is that people crumble mentally with age, and that the older you are, the dottier. But 78 per cent even of over-80s do not suffer from any form of dementia.

Let us not be mistaken about this. The fact that 22 per cent do suffer from dementia amounts to a million tragic victims, just as 13 per cent of over-65s being unable to move outdoors readily is a grave social issue. This is not whitewashing, but it is a matter of perspective.

The lesson is that you should begin with the stance that they are alright, that they are, so to speak, normal – and then adapt according to degrees, if any, of ill health and impairment, some of which may or should be temporary.

Avoid labels

No two people are alike. What should be recognised is that the two labels – "dependent" and "independent" – are not, in practice, quite so definite in composition. In some respects, the "severely dependent" person might be fiercely independent, and rightly so, insisting on this or that personal need.

A "reasonably independent" person, on the other hand, might be temporarily incapacitated or be absolutely dependent in one aspect of lifestyle. In the end, the blurring is such that it is much safer to take each client on his or her own terms as an individual.

Retirement

Many more people survive beyond 60 to enjoy another swathe of, one hopes, pleasant years. It is interesting to note that getting to 60 is the key. If you had arrived at 60 years of age in 1901, you could, on average, have expected another 13 or 14 years were left to you. If you reach 60 now, your anticipation might be of 15 or 16 years. Those are the male figures: females did and do somewhat better: but the point is the same. There's not that much difference. It's about survival.

Now, with earlier retirement, many, many people have a relatively long post-work span of life. Some people are retired for as long as they have worked.

This means, in turn, that clients crossing the threshold into retirement have increasingly spent a long time "at leisure". They are not coming to you direct from work, as would have sometimes happened in the past, nor equally, from completion of the happy chores of parenthood. Their children, did they exist, will be grown-up and away, and their jobs, did they have one, long ago over.

This raises an important issue. You should understand that, over the past years, the involvement of retired people in what might be called "constructive" activities (sports and pastimes, educational and recreational concerns) has been remarkably low. People take retirement all too seriously. They retire. They withdraw. They do very little. Don't be surprised if they are not eager for joining in any opportunities for activity you may offer. Many have been, in a word "counter-institutionalised": they have been ingrained into a lonely and negative lifestyle.

Choice and opportunity

Opportunities is the operative word. If one is a believer in giving maximum dignity and independence to older people then the critical thing is choice. Old people must choose to do this or that. If, acting with all the sensitivity to their previous perhaps negative background and offering the most tastily tempting of chances, the person still hands you the frozen mitt of refusal, that is her or his right.

If they do not want to do keep fit (to improve and maintain their physical suppleness), if they do not want to join in the quiz about World War II (designed to keep them mentally alert), if they do not want to create an Easter bonnet and process in an Easter parade (in the interests of social cohesiveness) so be it. They have made an informed choice, offered proper opportunities, and that is their civic right.

That entails the need for as much consultation as possible with clients. As far as possible, they should make the decisions, either the individual ones, like when to take a bath, or the collective ones, like who to vote for in a general election or participating in tenants association committees.

They are not children

There is a tendency to see normal ageing as a decline rather than a continuation. But frailty and weakness are not vices. Unconsciously, sometimes consciously, some treat very old people as children, as being in their "second childhood". This too has its attractions, but unluckily it is misleading. In any event, people do not always treat children as if they were "normal" and human: they do patronise them and assume responsibility for their rights; at worst, they humiliate them.

When this is applied to equally normal older people, the insult is compounded, for here are experienced veterans of life, who have grappled doughtily with all kinds of social problems, and who have perhaps remained resilient in the face of hammerblows – losing spouse, friends, income; suffering pain, hurt and indignity – each of which would floor many "ordinary" individuals.

One observes the trait in the forced ebullience with which older people are sometimes approached: in the use of forenames and endearments in a discourteously familiar way; in the presumption of decisions; in entering rooms without knocking; and in a score of tiny ways. By all means develop a close and warm if not sentimental (they are not "family") relationship, but do not assume it before it

occurs, any more than you would in the work place with a forty-year-old or in the local tennis club with a thirty-year-old.

Saints and sinners

Old people are normal. They are saints and sinners; more usually, mixtures of both. Some are cantankerous and quarrelsome and bloody nuisances, not because they are old, but because they probably always were. Old age does not confer a second childhood, and it does not convert to a benign mellowness. There will be rows. There will be good times, and bad.

The acid test is: would you like to receive the same type of care and attention that you are giving? The rule of thumb is sometimes said to be: do you look after the clients as you would look after your own mother? That's fine, but another question must be put: have you, as a person, the self-critical faculty which enables you to assess how well or badly you did or do look after your own mother. For a kick-off, did or do you *like* your own mother?

This is important. Please be honest. Care is about the whole person, not just about washing that bit or bandaging this bit. It is about enabling the full person to be as free, independent and yes, as happy as possible.

We should emphasise the old saying that every age has its compensations. This is very true. It should be the aim of the care assistant to help guarantee that each client's compensations are entirely realised.

NVQ Levels 2 & 3 Core Units
O Promote equality for all individuals.
Z1 Contribute to the protection of individuals from abuse.
W2 Contribute to the ongoing support of clients and others significant to them.
U4 Contribute to the health, safety and security of individuals and their environment.
U5 Obtain, transmit and store information relating to the delivery of a care service.

CHAPTER 12

Caring for people with mental health difficulties

Tim Martin

• A different, rewarding role for the care assistant • The skills you need – perception, communication, observation • How to build up a helpful, therapeutic relationship • Sharing information • Working as a team • Wider responsibilities

Caring for individuals suffering from mental health difficulties can be an interesting and rewarding area in which to work. One of its most interesting aspects is its "mystery". Mystery because unlike most other conventional health and social care needs it deals with often unseen, unmeasurable and inexplicable phenomena.

Popular public perceptions of mental health care are often gained from films such as *One Flew Over The Cuckoo's Nest* or *Silence of the Lambs*, where workers only leave the protection of offices to tighten the buckles of straitjackets on dangerous aggressive patients.

This notion was and is still reinforced by the older mental asylums which were built away from communities, and hidden behind walls. Fortunately such images of mental health care bear no resemblance to present-day reality.

Today most individuals with mental health difficulties receive treatment, care and support while remaining in their own home. Such people may appear to be very ordinary and act in a very normal way, particularly to the inexperienced eye. Discovering each individual's particular needs and responding to them with warmth and understanding, is the challenge for care staff.

Learning to cope with life

Each of us is a unique individual, genetically produced by parents, developed through a unique series of life experiences, and living in a unique life situation. So each of us reacts uniquely to the difficulties life inevitably brings.

Most of us are fortunate: we have the capacity to learn to cope with many difficult situations, and move successfully through life. The broadest definition of a person with mental health difficulties could be, an individual who fails to cope with their life situation.

Community Mental Health Services now offer a whole range of services, any number of which can be combined to tailor a specific package of care to treat the individual in their life situation.

In many areas the focus of these services is in local Mental Health Resource Centres. These facilities provide a base for teams of mental health staff from an assortment of professions offering a variety of skills; and a pleasant environment in which services can be offered away from the old fashioned institutions. Services can range from formal group psychotherapy, to informal drop-ins and coffee mornings.

From such centres individuals are offered "packages" of psychiatric care designed by the multi-professional team to meet their needs. This system is formalised as the Care Programme Approach to care.

The care programme approach is designed to ensure that each individual is assessed and reviewed by their care team regularly. From their assessment the team then decides what care or support the individual requires, and who is the best person or service to deliver each component of that care. The care team also nominate a named individual (key worker), to ensure that the care is coordinated before the next review date.

This does not mean the key worker must do everything, rather that it is their responsibility to coordinate the efforts of others, and establish if something hasn't, or can't be done, and why not, and report back to the care team as needed.

A care assistant will not be allocated as key worker in order to implement the care package. Key workers may be of any health care profession but are often Community Psychiatric Nurses, who are generally regarded as the backbone of community psychiatric care. Each carries a caseload of clients with mental health needs, whom they visit regularly, offering support and treatment, and monitoring their condition.

Your role

Stigma and public ignorance lead many people to believe mental illness is inevitably dangerous and incurable, and that society should be protected from mentally ill people. Your role in reality, as a care assistant, is much less sensational. In order to help someone, you must first begin to understand them as an individual, and learn the nature of their difficulties.

Without the luxury of visible signs and symptoms or advanced technology to investigate and monitor mental health needs, members of the caring team have to rely on their own personal skills to gain the essential information. This is not always easy in any situation, but can be particularly difficult when working with someone in their own home, their own territory, where you are a guest who *may* be shown only what your host wishes you to see. The vital skills you need are described under the headings that follow.

Perception

Perception is a key part of our lives. We are constantly receiving information through our senses, and taking action based on this information. Often this "data-analysis" is done so often we are not consciously aware we are doing it. How many times have you completed a task or activity, then when you stop and think back, you cannot remember the details of the task – it has become automatic.

To collect and interpret information from clients, it is important to be very aware of your perceptions. Seemingly unimportant remarks or changes in behaviour or appearance can give clues to an individual's difficulties and needs.

And of course this is a two-way process. It is just as important for you to be aware of how you are perceived by others. Clients are just as capable of picking up clues about our thoughts. It is impossible for us to like or relate well to everyone!

Communication

Communication is the most important component of mental health care. Your aim is to understand the individual, and effective communication with them is the best way to achieve that understanding.

Verbal communication

Talking and asking questions is an obvious method of finding things out, but it takes thought and practice to be effective.

Apart from considering the content of a conversation, we must also learn to understand other verbal cues such as the tone of voice, volume and word emphasis – all of which help to build up the true meaning of what is being said.

We may say one thing, while meaning or thinking something completely different. This can be either intentional or unconscious, but by carefully listening to the *way* things are said as well as *what* is said, we can learn much.

Non-verbal communication

Your understanding and awareness of the ways people communicate without words, is crucial. For example, eye contact is central to conversation: avoiding eye contact suggests mistrust, but too much can be threatening. Eye level is also important: physically looking up to someone can feel threatening (to you), looking down on someone can suggest dominance. Try to position yourself so that your eyes are on a level with those of the person with whom you are talking.

Observation

Aspects of an individual's behaviour give the observer vital clues to their inner thoughts and feelings, that may in turn be essential to understanding their difficulties or successfully delivering care.

Position: This may tell us a good deal. Is the person choosing to distance themself from others, sitting away in a corner? Perhaps they are feeling low or unworthy? Conversely, are they invading others' personal space, looming over them? Perhaps they are angry or frustrated?

Posture: A "closed" posture, for example sitting facing away from others with arms and legs crossed, suggests a disinterest in or fear of communication. Whereas sitting facing someone with arms and legs uncrossed may suggest a willingness for approach or involvement.

Appearance: We automatically infer a lot of information from the way a person looks, and this can influence what we expect of them and how we behave towards them if we are not careful. We might assume, for instance, that someone who is scruffy or dishevelled would lack motivation in other aspects of their life, whereas someone in a smart suit might be assumed competent and efficient. Both assumptions could be hopelessly inaccurate and misleading.

Interaction with environment: The way a person behaves in their environment gives clues. Someone smashing window panes is obviously disturbed with problems that need addressing immediately. But a different individual who sits staring at the wall may have equally pressing needs.

The above pointers are given as examples for guidance only. Each individual is unique, so to have any meaning an observation must be made and considered in context. A certain amount of knowledge and understanding of the individual is essential in order to judge what significance the observed activity has for them.

Rapport

To begin to build a helpful, therapeutic relationship with the client, the care assistant has to put all the above techniques into practice and work towards a mutual understanding, or "rapport". This is essential if you are to help them, because not many people are willing to share their difficulties with someone they consider to be a stranger.

You must be patient in your attempt to build a rapport. Remember that the client's situation and condition may well make them feel threatened and mistrustful of others. Try to "read" the situation and non-verbal clues to choose the best times to approach the client, and "read" the client's reactions to evaluate whether they are open and receptive to your efforts. If the client is becoming hostile or angry for instance, might it be better to withdraw and try again at another time?

In conversation it is better to have an honest, open approach to the client. Showing the client that you have *empathy* toward them is important. Empathy means showing you care about how they feel, and are willing to try to understand their situation, rather than *sympathy* which may be seen as condescending.

Be reliable

Being reliable is very important. It is very easy to promise to do something for a client, particularly if you are busy at the time, and because you might have a further twenty clients to think about, you forget to do it. The client however might have nothing else to think about but your promise, which could become very significant to them as a consequence.

A little thing (to you) such as taking someone to the shop at a certain time, might become central to their day. Failure to be reliable could have severe repercussions on your relationship. Don't make promises you might not be able to keep.

Professional boundaries

A successful rapport can often be a difficult balance to achieve. Your role is to get to know the person, develop an understanding and empathy for them, allow them to begin to know and trust you, and offer your services as a non-judgemental "friend". All this while always maintaining a professional overview of the relationship and situation.

Confidentiality of information is important, but care must be taken to acknowledge the boundaries within which you are working. It is important that you share information with other care workers, for the client's benefit in terms of consistency and continuity, and for your own benefit to ensure that you have the support and supervision of others and maintain a balanced perspective of the situation. Over-involvement and lack of supervision and support can be damaging to all concerned.

Sharing information

An important part of building rapport is developing trust. You should always endeavour to keep the client informed of what is happening to and around them. This means taking the time to explain actions and procedures to them in language they can understand, and encouraging their questioning and involvement in their own care process.

Remember you are likely to be the main contact between the client and the care system, so the client may ask you anything. It is important that you make sure you *can* answer the question before you try. Details of their illness or treatment for example are better explained by a qualified nurse or doctor. In some rare instances there may be information that the client should not be told (for example the telephone number of relatives). The golden rule should be, if you are in *any* doubt you must check with your supervisor.

Records and "hand-overs"

Information must flow throughout the care team. To ensure consistency and continuity of care, each member of that team needs to know what is going on. This means keeping effective records, and having regular "hand-overs" to exchange information between all those involved with the client's care. It will be up to the client, their key worker (or named nurse) and their care team to discuss and decide what should be divulged to non-professional carers and relatives.

Working as a team

It is important to remember you are part of a team. The care assistant's role within that team is a crucial one. You are generally the person who spends the most time with clients, and so you have access to the most information about individuals. Qualified staff are generally responsible for clients' care, upkeep of records, liaising with relatives and other professionals, but they have many constraints upon their time, and must rely on care assistants for a good deal of "hands-on" care. Therefore it is imperative that care assistants share their experiences, thoughts and feelings with the qualified staff.

Points to remember

1. Mental health care is concerned with addressing the needs of unique individuals.

2. Successful care is based on the care assistant's ability to understand and communicate effectively with their clients.
3. Good observation skills are crucial in mental health care.
4. Non-verbal communication skills are essential to good communication.
5. Communication with other staff, and teamwork, are fundamental to good care.
6. Care workers must remember their responsibilities to all others in the care process.

Suggested further reading

Manwatching by Desmond Morris, Triad Granada 1977.
The Naked Ape by Desmond Morris, Cape 1967.
Social Interaction by M.Argyle, Methuen 1978.
Stigma by I.Goffman, Penguin 1968.

NVQ Levels 2 & 3 Core Units
O Promote equality for all individuals.
Z1 Contribute to the protection of individuals from abuse.
U4 Contribute to the health, safety and security of individuals and their care environment.
U5 Obtain, transmit and store information relating to the delivery of a care service.

Level 2 Core Unit
W2 Contribute to the ongoing support of clients and others significant to them.

Level 3 Core Units
Z8 Support clients when they are distressed.
Y2 Enable clients to make use of available services and information.

Level 2 Domiciliary Support
Y1 Enable clients to manage their domestic and personal resources.
W8 Enable clients to maintain contacts in potentially isolating situations.
U1 Contribute to the maintenance and management of domestic and personal resources.

CHAPTER 13

Confusion and dementia

Alan Crump

*• What is confusion? • What is dementia? • The progress of dementia
– changes in understanding, personality and behaviour • Building up a
relationship of trust and respect • The right approach – clear communication,
reducing frustration and risks• The value of activities*

Caring for people with dementia is one of the most challenging areas of work. It can be both physically and mentally demanding, and at times it may feel that there are few rewards for your commitment, skill and patience. However, as a care assistant you have a key role to play in working with people with dementia. With the right attitude and approach you can make all the difference in their care. It may well be your efforts that allow someone to stay in their own home rather than move to a residential or nursing home.

What is confusion?

Confusion is a very broad term used to describe a situation where someone is unable to understand or function at the level you would normally expect of them. A person may not remember names, faces or previously well-known places. They may lose track of time or not understand simple information.

Some people may become very anxious, believing there is a plot against them by their relatives or carers. Others become withdrawn and isolated. "Confusion" is not a single condition; rather there is a whole set of different behaviours which might be associated with someone who is confused.

We all get confused

There are times when we all get confused. We walk into a new building or a different street and think that an office or shop is to the left and end up getting lost and confused. All of us forget important information at some time. A name of a friend, an item from the shopping list or a special appointment.

Illness can make people confused, both young and old. Severe influenza, a knock on the head, extreme anxiety or some medicines can cause some temporary confusion.

People can also become confused when they get chest infections, urine infections or heart problems. Again these periods of confusion are short and can be easily treated. An older person who suddenly becomes confused will probably have a condition which is easily treated.

For others, and for example people with AIDS, there is no cure. The dementia gets progressively worse and the person becomes more dependent.

As a care assistant you will get to know clients well, and you will be able to spot and report any sudden unexplained changes. Your knowledge of the person will be essential. With appropriate treatment the suddenly confused older person will return to the able and orientated person that you know.

However for some people, those who have dementia, confusion is something that they and all those around them have to live with every day of their lives.

What is dementia?

Dementia is a term which describes a decline in the ability to think clearly and remember accurately. This decline results in a reduced ability to care for yourself and sometimes involves changes to your personality. The outcome of all the changes to the person with dementia lead to them being "confused".

Confusion can take many forms. A person may show a range of behaviours or special needs. Although there may be some similarities, each person will have different losses and different abilities. Just as there is no condition which defines confusion there is no set of behaviours which defines dementia.

The progress of dementia

In the early stages of dementia, periods of confusion may be only short or they may involve only minor lapses in concentration or forgetfulness. Often the changes will only be noticed when one looks back and is able to see a pattern of certain behaviours.

It is important to remember that if someone forgets a name or an address this does not necessarily mean they have dementia. We all forget things and occasionally we all do unusual things. Being old is not the same as having dementia. Only five per cent of people over 65 have dementia. This only rises to twenty per cent of people over 80. The following are some behaviour changes that are common in dementia:

Memory loss
Memory loss will be most apparent at first with events and information that is recent. Forgetting that the kettle is on the stove. Losing important documents that were put into a "safe" place. Perhaps forgetting that they have just eaten and starting again, or asking the same question over and over again.

The usual pattern is that memories which are deeply embedded in the memory are the last to be lost. A person may have a very poor memory for the last thirty years, perhaps forgetting that a dearly loved spouse has died, but may have a very clear image of their early years of life.

Loss of understanding and reasoning
A person with dementia will begin to lose the ability to understand what is going on around them. For instance they may not see the importance of washing or dressing. They may not understand the need to have regular meals. If they go into shops they may make rash decisions, such as buying dog food when they do not have a dog!

People with dementia may be at risk when crossing busy roads. They may not understand the danger involved. On a cold day they may not realise it would be sensible to wear a coat outside.

Normal decision-making is altered. The ability to hold several ideas at the same time becomes increasingly difficult and decision making is frustrating.

Restlessness and agitation

A person with dementia may begin to show signs of being restless. This restlessness may have no specific cause, and cannot be fully explained. They may wander around the house or garden without any apparent aim. Attempts to prevent them pacing may be met with anger and resentment. This restlessness may mean that their sleep pattern is altered, perhaps sleeping little at night and napping during the day. Carers at home may find this aspect the most difficult to manage.

Changes to the personality

A person with dementia may seem to have large changes in their personality. They may seem obstinate where once they were cooperative and helpful. This may be as a result of the individual's desire to keep things as they are and not change anything, because this feels safer to them. They may become impatient and a little self-centred where once they were tolerant and generous.

They may start to depend upon one person for a sense of security, and become very anxious when that person is away. The person with dementia may develop ideas that someone is trying to harm them or steal from them. These ideas can become increasingly real for the individual and very difficult to change. Caring for a person with such strongly held ideas can be very difficult.

Physical and verbal aggression

The frustration and anxiety of the person with dementia can sometimes spill over into aggression. This might be shouting or strong language. Very occasionally it could result in physical blows. All these events may be completely out of the previously reported character of the patient. This can be particularly worrying for relatives.

Mood

Changes in mood are also possible, especially in the early stages of dementia. A person may seem distant and quiet. They may talk of dying and seem in low spirits. The person may realise that all is not as it should be and this may cause a great deal of distress. This kind of distress or depression may respond very well to medication. It will certainly respond well to warmth and genuine concern.

Loss of independence

Some people with dementia may slowly lose ability to do the normal everyday activities like washing, dressing, preparing and eating food and using the toilet. It may also affect activities like walking and speaking. As the illness progresses the abilities of the person with dementia decline to the point where they need help with every aspect of normal living.

A trusting relationship

The most important principle when working with a person who has dementia, is to limit their confusion or frustration. As a care assistant you may have to respond to a person who at times will believe they are living 30 years ago, and who believes they can cope without any help from "strangers".

The main aim of your care should be to develop a trusting relationship. A trusting relationship will mean that every other area of care will be that much easier.

Developing a trusting relationship is not easy. You may have to compete with some fixed ideas – for example they may believe you are stealing from them. Sometimes it is really difficult not to feel hurt and defensive. This kind of response creates frustration and even more feelings of insecurity. It will make every aspect of your care that much more difficult.

Patience

There are times when people will test your patience to its very extreme. Rushing and being impatient are counter-productive. There will always be a more positive response if your care is measured, calm and patient.

Tolerance

Some of the behaviours of the person appear quite irrational. Some individuals do things, say things and believe things that are very unusual. It may be strong language. It may be inappropriate sexual advances. It may be severe frustration or aggression aimed at you personally. You may be the person who takes all the blame. The least helpful response would be for you to become angry or frustrated with the person who is confused (see also chapter 20).

Sometimes you will have to step back for a few moments and "count to ten" in order to continue. This is something everyone has to do at times. Your tolerance in extreme situations will develop as you start to understand the frustrations of the individual with whom you are working.

Understanding and knowledge

Understanding and knowledge come with time, and help to build up the relationship. It helps a great deal if you try to understand the situation from the client's point of view. Try to feel the way they feel. We can never truly know what it is like to have dementia. However, with some knowledge of the condition, likely behaviours and causes, if we try to understand we can perhaps sense their

frustration, their pain, loss and distress.

Sensitivity

Sensitivity is not the same as being very caring. It is about doing the right things at the right times.

If a person with dementia was crying, a "caring" person might say "Oh, don't worry, it will all be all right". This is obviously not true, however, and could be called insensitive. The sensitive person would try and understand the frustration or the distress, and would not dismiss the feelings being expressed.

The "caring" person might see someone struggling with shaving or washing and do it for them. This might save time but would take away the fragile independence of the person with dementia. The sensitive person would offer time, encouragement and support.

Taking risks

Similarly, a "caring" person might restrict someone's ability to move around because of a feeling that they are at risk. This will keep them safe but may take away one of the most important freedoms that remains. Sometimes in promoting safety we end up by promoting lethargy and helplessness. The sensitive person would weigh up the risks to find the most appropriate solution.

Humour

This does not mean deliberate attempts to make someone feel small by laughing at them. It is about always being able to see the lighter side. Humour can be used to build relationships. Laughing with people develops understanding and shared feelings. Working with people who have dementia can sometimes seem very hard without much feedback. Watching someone smile and smiling with them can add something to the

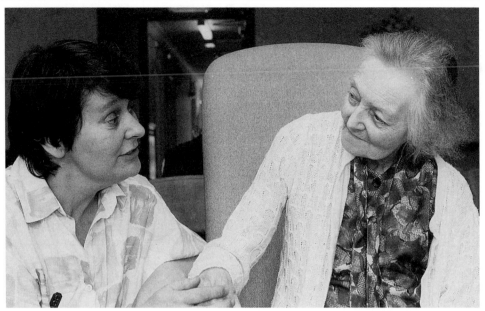

The main aim of your care should be to develop a trusting relationship. This will make every other area of care that much easier.

relationship that could not be offered in any other way.

Respect
When all the other qualities set out above are brought together, then the final quality will shine through. Respect comes when you can accept the person just as they are. It is the quality that is most difficult to define but which is crucial in building up a working relationship with the person with dementia.

The right approach

It is important to remember that a confused person will perform at their best when they are relaxed and free of frustration. To help with this you could consider the following:

Communication
At all times this needs to be as clear as possible. Avoid saying things in a complex way; keep sentences short. Use the same language that the individual uses:

if he says TV for television then use TV, if he uses bathroom to talk about the toilet then you should say bathroom.

If you have said something that is important and does not appear to have been understood, repeat it. Perhaps use simpler words. When the individual says they understand, get them to repeat it back to you in order to check. Many of the frustrations and anxieties for the person with dementia come from misunderstanding information.

Always bear in mind the use of a hearing aid or spectacles. Make sure the batteries are fresh and the ear piece is free of wax. Clean spectacles. These could vastly help in any aspect of communication. (See also chapter 5, Talking and listening.)

Names
How you address someone is important. If you call everyone "Gran" or "Dear" this will not show any respect or sensitivity. People have preferred names and

titles. Using these will show that you have thought about what you are doing. It gives the impression that the person to whom you are talking really counts. Nicknames and terms like "Sweetie" or "Lovey" are patronising, and the person may not understand that you are talking to them.

Avoiding confrontation

When working with a confused person never confront them with painful truths or harsh realities. Confrontation will cause anxiety and distress for the person with dementia. It will make your job that much more difficult.

If an individual talks about his deceased wife as though she were alive it is insensitive to confront him with the painful truth that she is dead. It would be more appropriate to talk about his feelings – how he is missing her.

Staying calm

Being calm is important. Staying calm will give you the best chance of persuading them, for example, to get washed or dressed. If they are very angry, and perhaps you have to change soiled clothing, then calmness remains the most appropriate approach. Often in these circumstances a "running commentary" will help, telling the confused individual what you are doing as you do it. Your unhurried and patient approach will show that you still care.

Making the environment less confusing

It is important that a person with dementia is given every chance to be as independent as possible for as long as possible. The home in which someone lives will be a familiar place but as their memory fails, even a familiar environment can become confusing and frightening. A person might forget the location of the toilet, or their bedroom. A simple sign on the door might be all a person needs to prompt them.

Reducing some of the risks

As a frequent visitor to the place where they live, you will be aware of some of the problem areas. Perhaps in the kitchen, where a change of cooker would improve safety. A change in the heating system from coal to an electric bar heater. some simple changes will make the home less confusing and may mean that a person can stay at home longer (see chapter 14).

Creating a supportive routine

A regular routine during the day will help reduce confusion. It can help to make people feel more secure because they know what is going to happen. At these times clear information is important to reduce anxiety, for instance if the usual care assistant is sick and you have to take their place.

We all have routines, but these are very individual to ourselves, such as the times that we eat, the soap and toothpaste we use, and so on.

Creating a routine can be helped by making your visits at more or less the same time. Clocks in the house should be clear and correct. Meal times should occur at approximately the same time each day. Tablets and medicine should be kept to a minimum but if an individual has a good routine then remembering to take them will be made easier.

Supporting carers

It is important to remember that by supporting a carer you will be helping to keep someone in their own home for longer (see chapter 23, Carers and relatives).

Activities

Each person with dementia is a unique individual. They have their own likes and dislikes. They have a history. They may have been a great one for putting on their best clothes every Wednesday and going out to the local dance or club. They may have been the one that sat at home and watched all the soaps curled up with the gas fire on and a good book. They may have been the one that was the respected shop steward, always out at meetings in smoke-filled rooms.

When considering activity we often think immediately of games or making something or being part of a group. We should remember that for some the act of getting up, choosing clothes and dressing is a major and important activity in itself. If we can value the normal activities and make them special, then finding meaningful pastimes for people with dementia will be that much easier.

The really important point to remember is that different people need and enjoy different types of activity. Not all men enjoy football and not all women enjoy knitting. It would be a dull world indeed if we all enjoyed the same things. The message therefore is to get to know the people who you care for and discover their interests. A knowledge of someone's previous background and history will give clues to what they will enjoy doing now.

By working with people and helping them to do the activities which give them pleasure however small (or large) you will really make a difference. Sometimes it is difficult to see how our care can make a difference but by making activity a regular event, the difference quickly becomes apparent.

Points to remember

1. We all get confused. Just because someone is confused it does not necessarily mean they have dementia.
2. Sudden confusion is usually the result of a treatable condition.
3. Dementia is a condition which results in a gradual decline in the ability to think clearly and remember accurately.
4. The qualities you should try to develop include:
• Patience
• Tolerance
• Understanding
• Sensitivity
• Humour
• Respect.
5. The right approach will help you to develop a good working relationship with the patient. Bear in mind the following areas:
• Good clear communication.
• Using appropriate names and titles.
• Avoiding confrontation.
• Staying calm.
• Making the home less confusing.
• Reducing some of the risks.
• Creating a supportive routine.
• Supporting relatives.

NVQ Levels 2 & 3 Core Units
O Promote equality for all individuals.
U4 Contribute to the health, safety adn security of individuals and their environment.
U5 Obtain, transmit and store information relating to the delivery of a care service.

Level 2 Core Unit
W2 Contribute to the ongoing support of clients and others significant to them.

Level 3 Core Units
Z3 Contribute to the management of aggressive and abusive behaviour.
Y2 Enable clients to make use of available services and information.

Level 2 Direct Care
Z6 Enable clients to maintain and improve their mobility.

Level 2 Domiciliary Support
W8 Enable clients to maintain contacts in potentially isolating situations.

CHAPTER 14

Safety, accidents and first aid

Jill Cowley

• Recognising risk factors • Infants and pre-school children • School age children
• Adults and older people • Principles of first aid • Action in an emergency
• Cardio-pulmonary resuscitation of adults

The place in which we live and the environment in which we work can greatly affect our health. We can't directly control every aspect of the world around us, but we can each take individual responsibility for maintaining safety in our immediate environment and for looking after the safety of our clients and colleagues, and our own wellbeing.

All care staff have a responsibility to give appropriate advice on safety and accident prevention, and to know the correct First Aid measures and carry them out quickly. These are key factors to ensure that people remain free from harm, or that injuries are reduced and recovery is hastened.

Recognising risk factors

It is important that you can recognise potentially harmful situations or people considered most at risk. As a care assistant you need to be extra vigilant in recognising potential dangers and reporting these to a qualified member of staff.

Care assessments need to highlight unsafe situations, and care plans need to include your aim to raise your clients'

awareness of risks and promote their ability to avoid them. If, during your work, you encounter someone who has had an accident you may need to give First Aid or help.

The Government report *Health of the Nation* provides targets for reducing accidents and illness, disability or death that may arise as the result of accidents. People who are most at risk include children, older people and those who may have a physical or mental illness. This provides a useful framework for considering some situations that you might encounter in people's homes and elsewhere in the community.

Infants and pre-school children

Babies and infants under one year have not usually had the opportunity to learn about or understand what can be potentially dangerous. They are totally dependent upon their carers, parents or others to protect them from harmful situations.

Accidents are the commonest cause of death in pre-school children. You can help avoid these dangers by reminding parents and guardians of any risks to safety. Your own experience of family members can also be used to help to reinforce any advice given by qualified members of staff.

Choking and suffocation

Infants soon learn how to pick up small objects and how to place these in their mouths. Small objects such as beads, small toys and food such as peanuts, should be kept out of reach. Large, soft, age-appropriate toys, without plastic eyes, nose or mouths that meet safety standards should always be encouraged. Babies should never be left alone with a bottle. They should always be propped upright in the cot or chair to ensure that they are not at risk of rolling over and choking.

If children are allowed to play with string or ribbons (often tied to dummies and gloves to prevent them being lost) these might accidentally become wound around their neck. Polythene or plastic bags should always be kept out of reach to prevent children placing them over their heads and suffocating.

Falls

As small babies and infants learn how to rock and crawl about they are at risk of falling off beds and chairs if they are unsupervised. Stair gates are important to prevent infants from climbing and falling. Some equipment designed specifically for small children, such as baby walkers and bouncing chairs, can also be dangerous if they tip over or become caught on unprotected fires or radiators.

Special locks can be fitted to windows and doors to prevent these opening too widely. Some bannister rails on landings and stairs can also be wide enough for a child to fall through.

Protective helmets and elbow and knee pads can help to prevent fractures, and particularly head injuries, when children are learning to ride bicycles and skate boards. Young children should always be supervised when cycling to stop them straying into the path of oncoming traffic.

Burns and scalds

As infants learn how to stand and grasp objects the dangers of pulling kettle flexes or saucepans are increased. Cooker guards may need to be used, or handles and flexes kept well out of reach and positioned towards walls.

The temperature of bath water should always be checked before bathing and infants should never be left alone in the bath even if they look well supported.

Fixed fire guards need to be placed on electric, gas and coal fires. Ovens can also become very hot and children need to be confined to play areas that do not place them at risk. Burns can also be caused by electricity. Special plugs can be used to prevent infants from placing their fingers in electric sockets.

Sunburn

Exposure to strong sunlight can cause sunburn in varying degrees with anything from redness and itching to burns with blisters and swelling. Burning can be increased by wind, salt, water or light reflected from sea and snow. Fair haired people burn more easily because they have less protection from skin pigment. People on certain types of medication may be more at risk of burning.

Encourage clients to use a high protection sun cream, especially on small children, and to reapply regularly, especially if they play in the sea or pool.

If affected, rest the child in the shade, and don't allow him to go into the sun again unless the burned areas are covered with light, loose clothing. Give him plenty to drink.

Mild sunburn can be soothed with calamine lotion or by bathing the child in cool water.

In cases of severe sunburn, do not burst the blisters. Obtain medical advice if the sunburn is distressing, and accompanied by headache, nausea, or fever.

Car safety

Babies and infants should always sit in the rear of cars, preferably in a special child seat with restraining seat belts. Most modern cars have a child lock facility that prevents the door from being accidentally opened from the inside.

Cuts

When infants start to walk and run, safety glass in low-level doors and windows is the best option. Special clear film can also be applied to prevent glass from splintering. Sharp knives and scissors need to be kept out of reach of children. They should be encouraged to remain seated if using pencils or eating lollipops with sharp sticks attached.

Poisoning

Medicines should always be kept locked away in child resistant containers. Alcohol, household cleaning chemicals, and garden chemicals also need to be kept in their original containers and locked away out of reach.

Drowning

Children can drown even in very shallow water. They need to be supervised while they are bathing or playing near water or garden ponds. Learning to swim can prevent children from drowning and also promote activity that will encourage them to remain fit and healthy.

School age children

Road traffic accidents

Road traffic accidents are the largest single cause of accidental death in school age children. Safe car travel and road safety are essential. Children are often unaccompanied on the streets at this age and road crossing safety is important. National campaigns, leaflets and posters are available to be displayed in schools, health centres and other community sites. Leaflets can be given to parents and children to reinforce road safety messages.

If children are cycling to and from school they need to be aware that lights and bright equipment are important to ensure that other road users can see them. Cycle helmets, protective clothing and courses in cycling proficiency need to be encouraged.

Poisoning

Alcohol and drugs can be very inviting to school age children who are ready to try out new things. Children may see "glue sniffing", drug use and smoking as a grown-up activity and wish to try it out for themselves. Children often feel compelled to join in with their friends and classmates.

Adults and older people

Road safety

Road traffic accidents cause most of the accidental deaths in older people. Illness and disability may make people less agile and reduced vision or hearing may mean that they are less able to judge distances accurately. Encouraging the use of designated crossings, and regular sight and hearing tests, can help reduce risks.

Falls

Many factors are responsible for falls. If older people sustain fractures because of a fall this may result in lengthy hospital admission, loss of independence and a loss of confidence in walking in the future. Preventing falls is one of the most important accident prevention roles with older people.

Food poisoning

Older people have a decreased resistance to bacteria that may be present in food. Food stored at the wrong temperature (either not hot enough or not cold enough) and incorrect cooking can easily help bacteria to multiply and affect the older person when it is consumed. Good food hygiene is essential to prevent accidental food poisoning.

Hypothermia

Hypothermia occurs when the body temperature falls below about 35 degrees Celsius. You should suspect hypothermia if you find a person unexpectedly ill or injured at home and the environment and weather is cold. Hypothermia is a common condition in the UK. It develops slowly and may not be noticed for several hours. The person may be shivering, have a loss of memory and poor judgement. When the temperature falls lower, the person may become blue (cyanosed) and the heart and blood pressure rates will fall, eventually leading to loss of consciousness. Feeling the abdomen (tummy) rather than hands and feet will give a better indication of hypothermia if this is the problem.

You will need to wrap the person in warm blankets, ensuring that you cover the head. The room should be gently heated and warm drinks can be given. Do not give alcohol as this reduces the body temperature. Emergency help should be summoned as soon as possible.

Prevention of hypothermia is the main aim. Older adults, babies and people with damage to the nervous system are at most risk. Advice on the need for hot drinks, at least one hot meal per day, and wearing several layers of clothes needs to be provided. Some people may be afraid of high heating and fuel bills and need financial help and advice.

Principles of First Aid

During your work, you may have to deal with an emergency until help arrives.

Universal precautions

Hepatitis B and HIV infection are carried in blood and these can be passed on to another person if blood enters their body through cuts in the skin. In an emergency, you should remember the risks and precautions that should be taken. Where possible, show the person how to apply First Aid themselves, such as applying pressure to a bleeding wound.

Disposable gloves may already be available in the client's home if dressings are being carried out. Alternatively, you may need to avoid contact with blood and fluids by using sufficient absorbent material, such as towels. If you do come into contact with blood, wash the affected area thoroughly under running water for at least ten minutes. Always report this to a qualified member of staff who will advise you on the local policy to follow.

To be absolutely safe, universal precautions should also apply to faeces, vomit, tears, saliva, sputum, sweat, nasal secretions and urine. Follow the advice and example of qualified staff.

Action in an emergency

Assess the situation calmly and quickly. First Aid is all about simple observation – for example skin colour, obvious bleeding, temperature, breathing and swelling or distortion of limbs – and simple but immediate action.

Don't place yourself in obvious danger from fires, toxic gases, chemicals, electricity or unsafe buildings and equipment. Always summon help. Calm the person and others who may be present. Do not give drinks or food, particularly alcohol, until you are certain that medical help is not required.

Collapse due to shock is a common feature of accidents. You need to check three things; airway, breathing and circulation.

• **Airway** – Check the mouth and nose to make sure that they are not blocked by the person's tongue, food, vomit or other foreign body. The safest way to maintain an

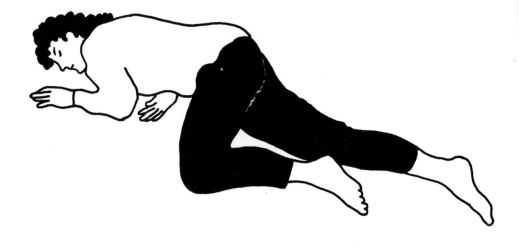

Fig 1. The recovery position – the safest way for an unconscious person to lie.

airway is to place the person on a hard surface in the recovery position (Fig 1). If you suspect any broken bones, neck or back injury, it may be safer not to move them, but clear the mouth and nose and check for breathing. See if you can rouse the person by asking them **loudly** to respond to you: "Jane – are you alright?"

• **Breathing** – Listen and look for signs or sounds of breathing. You could feel their breath on your face or see the person's chest rising and falling. Loosen any tight clothing around the person's neck and chest. Tilting the head back and holding the jaw forward will make sure that the airway is opened and that air can enter the lungs (Fig 2).

• **Circulation** – feel the person's pulse, either at the wrist or the carotid pulse at the side of the Adam's apple in the neck. If the person does not appear to be breathing, there is no pulse and they are unresponsive to your attempts to rouse them you may need to start cardio-pulmonary resuscitation.

Cardio-pulmonary resuscitation of adults

Breathing

Lay the person on their back on a firm surface. Tilt the head back and lift the jaw (Fig 2). Pinch the nostrils together, place your mouth securely over the person's mouth to create a seal, and breath into the mouth.

If your client has a tracheostomy (a breathing hole in the centre of the neck) it needs to be cleared and air blown into it.

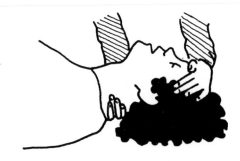

Fig 2. Preparing for mouth to mouth resuscitation: tilt the head back and lift the jaw.

Look to see if the chest is rising and falling. If breathing starts spontaneously after this has been carried out, place the person in the recovery position. Continue to observe them. Their skin should return to a lighter, more normal colour. Wait for help to arrive.

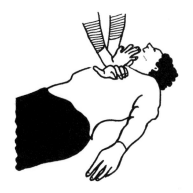

Fig 3. The correct position of hands for cardiac massage.

Circulation

If the heart has stopped, you will notice that the lips, tongue, ear lobes and finger nails may become bluish-grey in colour. The pupils of the eyes may be fixed and very large. If you cannot feel a pulse or hear a heartbeat you will need to start cardiac resuscitation.

Place the heel of one hand over the lower centre of the breastbone (one finger breadth below a line joining the nipples). Place the heel of the other hand on top, keeping the palms and fingers forward. With your arms straight, rock backwards and forward (Fig 3). Each time that you rock forward you will be compressing the chest and heart to stimulate the pumping action. If you are on your own repeat this fifteen times, stop, and then breath into the lungs twice. Keep going until help arrives or the person shows signs of responding. When a second person is present one should give five heart massages, then the other two breaths, then keep repeating the sequence.

With successful resuscitation the person's skin colour will look more normal, a carotid pulse will be felt and the pupils will look less dilated. If the person has stopped breathing, the heart may still be pumping. If the heart has stopped beating the breathing will certainly cease.

Special techniques for children are also taught and you should take advantage of any training offered.

Choking, suffocation and drowning

Choking may be recognised by the person having a coughing fit and being unable to breathe. Smacking the person smartly, three or four times between the shoulders can be used to try and dislodge any foreign body or use the Heimlich Manoeuvre (Fig 4). Infants can be held upside down by the legs and older children can be laid across the knees. A person who has been rescued from drowning needs to be placed in the recovery position (Fig 1) so that water can run freely from the lungs and mouth. The rules for cardio-pulmonary resuscitation should be followed.

Burns, scalds and electric shock

The aim of treating burns is to stop the burning, relieve pain, limit the swelling and reduce any risk of infection. If possible, flood the burn or scald with cool running water for at least ten minutes. Remove any jewellery from the injured area, as it may swell and be difficult to remove later. Never attempt to pull away clothing that is sticking to the skin. Cover the area with clean dry linen, gauze or a non-adherent dressing. Burns to the eye should be treated in the same way. Always refer clients for medical attention.

Burns caused by electricity occur where the current has entered or left the body and should be treated in the same way as any burn. Always make certain the electric-

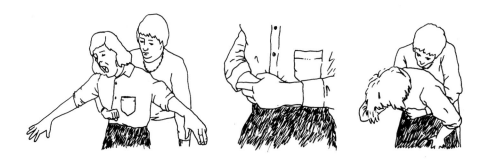

Fig 4. The Heimlich Manoeuvre. 1. Stand behind the choking victim and clench one fist, thumb towards her stomach. 2. Hold this fist tight with the other hand – it should be placed under the ribs, between the navel and breastbone. 3. Pull sharply inwards and upwards, three or four times (pushing the upper abdomen against the lungs to force air violently upwards).

ity supply has been switched off before attending to a person.

Cuts and bleeding

A small amount of blood can seem a lot worse than it is. Check the wound to make sure that no large splinters of glass, wood or other sharp materials are present. Pressure needs to be applied directly over the wound. If a foreign body is deeply embedded, apply pressure to the side of it.

Spurting, bright red blood will mean that an artery (vessel carrying blood being pumped from the heart) has been damaged. This is the most serious wound and must be treated, by applying pressure, as a priority.

Small cuts and abrasions need to be cleaned under a running tap or by pouring clean water over the area.

Internal bleeding is difficult to detect unless the person is vomiting blood. Keep the person still, warm and comfortable while you wait for help.

Poisoning

Poisons may accidentally enter the body by breathing fumes, absorption through the skin or stomach and puncturing of the skin.

If the person has inhaled a poison they need fresh air and assistance to sit in a position that helps them to breathe. If a poison has been swallowed, do not induce vomiting. Ask them what substances they have swallowed, or look around for any containers that may provide clues. Place them in the recovery position and seek medical help.

Anaphylactic shock

Anaphylactic shock can occur as the result of an insect sting or bite. Although rare, it can also occur when a client has eaten something or when a medicine has been given orally or via injection. The person quickly complains of a tight chest, has difficulty breathing and becomes blue (cyanosed) in colour. The pulse becomes rapid and their blood pressure will drop. This will eventually lead to collapse and respiratory or cardiac arrest.

Reassurance is essential. If a qualified member of staff is present they may be carrying and able to give injections of adrenaline. In addition all the rules of cardio-pulmonary resuscitation described above should be followed. Medical help should always be summoned immediately.

Afterwards

After administering any First Aid ensure that your client receives medical help. Report the signs, symptoms and care that you gave to a qualified member of staff. Do not leave the client until you are certain that you have done everything that you were able to, and that you have done your best.

Points to remember

1. Everyone needs to take individual responsibility for maintaining a safe environment and for looking after the safety of clients, colleagues and our own wellbeing.

2. Advice on safety, accident prevention, and knowing what First Aid actions to carry out in the event of an accident, are essential.

3. Acting quickly and appropriately in case of accidents are key factors to ensure that people remain free from harm, or that injuries are minimised and that recovery is hastened.

4. Care assessments need to highlight unsafe situations and care plans need to include the aim to raise your clients' awareness and promote their ability to avoid accidents.

5. People identified as at most risk include children, older people and those who have a physical or mental illness.

6. Take the opportunity to participate in any First Aid training and education.

Resources

British Red Cross Society
9 Grosvenor Crescent,
London. SW1X 7EJ
Tel: 071-235-5454

St. John's Ambulance Association
1 Grosvenor Cresent
London
SW1X 7ES
Tel: 071 235 5231

Royal Society for the Prevention of Accidents
Cannon House
The Priory, Queensway
Birmingham B4 6BS
021 200 2461
Department of Health (1992) *Health of the Nation: A Strategy for Health In England*. HMSO, London.

NVQ Level 2 & 3 Core Units
O Promote equality for all individuals.
U4 Contribute to the health, safety and security of individuals and their environment.
U5 Obtain, transmit and store information relating to the delivery of a care service.

Level 2 Core Unit
W2 Contibute to the ongoing support of clients and others significant to them.

Level 3 Core Unit
Y2 Enable clients to make use of available services and information.

CHAPTER 15

Practical care for people at home

Jennie Williams and Stuart Darby

• Assessing individual care needs • Care plans • Giving practical care
• Communication • Taking routine observations
• Aspects of personal care

Working as a care assistant in the community will involve giving practical care to people who are ill, have a disability or are recovering from illness. Some clients will live alone while others will have family and friends who also need support and help. Providing practical care involves assessing individual clients' needs, planning care in collaboration with them and other agencies, and finally providing practical help and recording any activities carried out.

Assessing individual needs

The Community Care Act now means that a coordinated approach must be taken by all community care workers to enable people to stay in their own home. Working with specialist services and other local and voluntary agencies is essential to planning and providing coordinated care which is acceptable to all concerned.

There are many different ways of organising care for people in their own homes. Qualified nurses, usually district nurses, are responsible for writing a care plan based on detailed assessments of each

client's health needs. All the members of the nursing team are expected to refer to this plan, which is usually kept in the client's own home. Other health and social service workers may share these notes. This helps to ensure that a coordinated approach to care is taken and that everyone understands the short and long term aims. The priority for care plans is that they should always be understood by the client and reflect what they want, as far as possible.

Care plans – first stage information

Care plans involve an initial assessment by a qualified member of staff who will interview, examine and observe the client for any existing or potential health needs.

Essential information includes the name, address and telephone number and date of birth of the client. The address and telephone number of a person to contact in an emergency and the name of the client's GP must also be included. The reason for referral, or diagnosed illness or disability may also be recorded. What the client understands about their condition is recorded as this helps to plan care that is realistic to their expectations.

Other types of information may include home conditions, toilet and washing facilities, steps and stairs that may be encountered and the names and numbers of other services involved. A general history of health problems will provide a picture for planning future care and meeting individual needs. This should also include the client's first language, their religious or cultural needs, their occupation and their recreational activities.

Care plans – second stage information

This involves systematically collecting and assessing data and recording routine observations. Routine observations (included below), are recorded so that any change in the person's condition can be monitored and matched against the first assessment. Other types of assessment may include:

Activity and movement: the use of walking aids or sticks, ability to move in bed, chair and around the home.

Rest and sleep: the length of time a person sleeps, where they sleep, if they use night sedation, if they need extra pillows or a bed cradle.

Nutrition and diet: including appetite, eating habits, food and drink likes and dislikes, any difficulty with swallowing, dehydration, malnutrition, weight loss or gain, nausea, vomiting, and mouth or denture care.

Elimination: bowel and bladder problems, urine testing, constipation or diarrhoea, access to toilet facilities, ability to dress/undress to use the toilet.

Breathing and circulation: difficulties with breathing, positioning for breathing, promoting blood circulation to all parts of the body by active movement, and prevention of pressure sores.

Pain: such as the location and degree of pain, and the method of coping with it.

Skin condition: dehydration, wounds, cuts, bruises, areas of the body at risk of damage from pressure, and pressure sores.

Emotional state: the client's own perception of their health, their ability to communicate and express their feelings or understand what is going on, and whether they are withdrawn, depressed, agitated, irritable, or confused and disorientated.

Care plans

A typical care plan is shown on p110. It will identify the date and any existing or potential problems that the client may have. Next to this will be the expected outcome or goal. The care plan will include details of what care should be given, when and by whom, to achieve these goals.

Progress sheets

A progress sheet may be available for you to complete and sign each time that you give care. This is an important record because it shows that you have been to see the client and carried out the necessary care. Care plans may include other specific documents to be signed, for example medicine administration charts and wound management charts.

Care plans are usually evaluated and revised regularly although this depends upon the needs of each client. This also gives clients the chance to evaluate their care and say whether things are getting better, remain the same or are getting worse. It will always be the responsibility of a qualified member of staff to evaluate and revise care plans.

Recording and reporting care

As a health care assistant you must be aware of the need to record any care you have given, and report any concerns or changes to a qualified member of staff. You should make these records before leaving the client's home. All records need to be legible, signed, and dated. You play a vital role in contributing to planning care

DATE	ACTUAL/POTENTIAL PROBLEM	AIM/EXPECTED OUTCOME	NURSING ACTION	PATIENT/CARER INPUT	SIGNATURE AND DATE OF EVALUATION
24th October 1994	1. Mrs Jones often has dribbling of urine due to condition.	Keep Mrs Jones continent and ask each week about satisfaction with management of incontinence.	a) Offer commode for use at night b) Encourage to use toilet regularly c) Wash, dry and apply cream to groin when Mrs Jones is wet.	Mrs Jones to use toilet regularly. Mr Jones will help with washing and applying cream. Commode by bed at night.	
	2. Mrs Jones has tendency to be constipated.	Bowels open every other day (normal pattern).	a) Encourage drinks b) Encourage fibre in diet – change to wholemeal bread c) Add bran to breakfast cereal.	Mrs Jones to ensure regular drinks. Mr Jones to look at fibre content of food when shopping.	
	3. Mrs Jones at risk of developing pressure sores.	Prevent pressure sores.	a) Ensure sheepskin in bed. b) Encourage to move position when sitting. c) Observe heels, sacrum and elbows and hips d) Encourage Vitamin C in diet through fresh fruit/fruit juice.	Mrs Jones to eat at least one piece of fruit each day.	
	4. Mrs Jones has difficulty sleeping.	Normal pattern 7-8 hours.	a) GP to prescribe night sedation b) Have last drink at 8pm to prevent need to use commode c) Ensure comfort – heat/cold.	Mr Jones to telephone GP. Mr Jones to arrange extra blankets.	

A care plan (extract above) identifies problems and goals of care, with details of the care that should be given to achieve these goals.

from your own observations or conversations with the client. You must ensure that you receive advice and support in carrying out your duties, particularly as you may spend much of your day working alone and will be required to plan your visits according to your client's needs.

Giving practical care

Your role in enabling people to remain at home will vary, but should only ever involve aspects of care for which you have been trained and feel competent to carry out. Some clients will always require a qualified member of staff and others will require a second person for support and assistance. On occasions you may need to ask the qualified member of staff to accompany you on a visit, if you are concerned about a client or an aspect of care that you have been asked to do.

When you are away from the work base, you should always know how to contact a qualified member of staff, either by bleep or client telephone number. It makes sense to always have money available to make a telephone call while out visiting.

Communication

Communication problems can be caused

by confusion, or misunderstanding speech, physical actions or body language. In situations where English is not the first language, it may be necessary for an interpreter to accompany you. Poor vision or hearing can contribute to poor communication and may make things worse.

There are many practical ways that you can help clients. Always wear a name badge and introduce yourself when you visit. This will help to ensure that the client feels confident about who you are and what you do. Writing your name on records or information sheets held by the client, along with a contact address and number, will enable them to feel secure about contacting you in the future.

Speak clearly, with a normal pitch, even when clients have hearing difficulties. Shouting does not help. Make sure that you are facing the client and have eye contact. You may want to touch as a part of your introduction if your client is blind or partially sighted but always explain what you are about to do in advance (see also chapter 5, Talking and listening).

If a client wears spectacles check that they are clean, and ensure that the room is well lit. If a hearing aid is used, make sure that it is switched on and working. It may need re-tubing or new batteries.

Your client may use a pendant security alarm, usually a small device worn around the neck or wrist, which can be activated in an emergency to call help. Make sure that they have it with them before you leave and check that the telephone is working and close to hand. Offer to switch on the radio or television if the client wishes. This can help them to keep in contact with the outside world, particularly if they live alone or if they are housebound.

Maintaining a safe environment
Ensuring safety in the home can be difficult because the home is not designed for nursing activities and is not a clinical area

– it is a place for living. It is important to ensure that any adaptations to ensure safety are negotiated with the client and that a homely environment is maintained.

You do have a responsibility to ensure your clients' wellbeing, your own safety, and protecting other members of staff who may also visit. The care that you give must not expose anyone to injury or unnecessary danger. The following list of examples show how you might be involved:
• helping clients to keep medicines stored safely (see chapter 19)
• performing minor dressings without introducing infection
• moving and transferring safely within the home (see chapter 17)
• reporting dangers such as faulty gas, electric or water systems
• reporting dangers to colleagues to prevent them from injuring themselves
• knowing when appliances, equipment or aids need maintenance, repair or replacement
• returning the client's keys to a locked key safe when you return to your work base.

Taking routine observations

Some clients may require routine observations or "vital signs" to be measured and recorded. These include pulse rate, temperature, blood pressure, samples of urine and finger prick blood testing.

Vital signs give important information about a client's state of health. They can be taken when a client is first assessed to provide a baseline for measuring any changes that may occur in the future. They may also be used to regularly monitor illness progression or improvement. You should be given clear instructions if you are told to act on any of the findings, other than simply reporting to a qualified member of staff.

Pulse rate

When the heart beats, an impulse is transmitted in a wave-like fashion into the arteries. This pulse can be measured by placing the first two fingers on the radial artery, found on the thumb side of the wrist. You should wait for five minutes before taking the pulse if the person has been taking active exercise. The pulse rate is counted for one full minute and the number of beats, rhythm of the beat and strength is noted.

A normal resting pulse should be between 60-80 beats per minute. The pulse rate may be faster (tachycardia) or lower (bradycardia) than normal.

There are many causes of a fast pulse rate. These include the need for the body to provide a greater supply of oxygen and energy to vital organs in the body; a reduced ability of the blood to carry oxygen; and heart disease where the heart rate increases to compensate for a weak or under functioning heart. A low pulse rate usually suggests irregular heart action. This may be caused by certain drugs and medicines but there are other causes.

Temperature

An oral thermometer is the most common way of measuring temperature when clients are able. At least fifteen minutes should elapse before taking a temperature if clients have been drinking or smoking. The thermometer should be cleaned, placed under the tongue and the mouth closed. After a minimum of three minutes a recording can be made. Normal temperature is approximately 37 degrees Celsius. A raised temperature may be caused by infection, pain, or a reaction to medicines. Examples of a low temperature commonly include Hypothermia (see p103) and poor circulation.

Blood pressure

Taking blood pressure is an important part of monitoring certain illnesses or the action of medicines. Blood pressure measurement requires special skills, teaching and practice. If you are asked to take and record a blood pressure make certain that you are competent. The vast majority of people, including doctors and nurses, need to practice many times before they can locate the specific pulse, hear the beat of the pulse and be certain of the peaks and troughs that they are recording. It is essential that you follow the correct procedure and technique.

Blood pressure is measured by an instrument known as a manometer. This consists of an inflatable cuff and a mercury column or dial that measures the pressure in the cuff. The cuff is placed around the upper arm and attached to the manometer. A stethoscope is placed over the brachial artery, found in the middle of the arm at the inside elbow joint. The cuff is pumped up slowly. The pressure in the cuff is now slowly released by turning a screw. When the thumping of the artery can be heard through the stethoscope, the pressure is read on the manometer. This is the systolic pressure. The pressure in the cuff is now further reduced until the thumping over the pulse dies away. This is the diastolic pressure. The systolic reading represents the maximum pressure of blood in the artery as the heart muscle contracts. The diastolic reading shows pressure as the heart muscle relaxes. Blood pressure is therefore recorded as the systolic over the diastolic, for example 120/90.

Blood pressure can rise as we get older. The normal systolic pressure in adults at rest averages from 110 to 150 millimetres of mercury (mmHg) on the manometer. The diastolic pressure averages between 60 and 85 mmHg. However, no two people are the same. If you are taught and asked to take and record blood pressure, you must record the results accurately and report to a qualified member of staff.

Urine testing

The client should be asked for a fresh sample of urine in a sterile container. A plastic "reagent strip" containing small patches of paper impregnated with chemicals is inserted into the urine. These patches will change colour and should be read according to the instructions on the container.

Common tests may indicate that the urine is too acid or alkali, which may influence the type of antibiotic to be used if a patient has an infection. Protein may be present if the client's kidneys are not functioning properly and ketones may be present if the client is dehydrated or malnourished. Blood in the urine may indicate a lower urinary tract infection, and a raised specific gravity will mean that the urine is very concentrated – commonly caused by lack of fluids and dehydration. The most common reagent strips are used to measure glucose (sugar) levels in people who have diabetes. A presence of glucose may indicate a change to the amount of insulin that they take or alterations to their daily diet. Always consult a qualified member of staff if the reading is not normal.

Finger prick blood testing

Finger prick blood testing for blood glucose (blood sugar) is usually taught to and undertaken by individuals who have diabetes. Some people however, are unable to manage alone and need assistance. Disposable gloves should be used for this technique.

The client should wash their hands, making certain that there is no soap residue. A plastic device that fits over a finger is fitted with a disposable pin. The finger or thumb is placed in the device and the trigger is released. This causes a small pin prick and allows a droplet sample of blood to be placed onto a plastic "reagent strip". The strip is read after a predetermined time. A normal blood glucose level should be between 3.5-7.5 millimoles of glucose per litre. You should always ensure that the pin and any materials in contact with the blood are disposed of correctly and safely. Always consult a qualified member of staff if the reading is below or above what you were told to expect.

Aspects of personal care

Helping clients to eat and drink

Encouraging clients to eat a healthy diet and reporting problems such as lack of appetite, difficulty chewing or swallowing is very important. We all need vital nutrients, proteins and carbohydrates so our bodies can function normally. If your client has a wound or pressure sore, it is even more important that their diet is sufficient in vitamins, zinc and other tissue repairing foods.

Ensuring that someone has had adequate fluids, about two to three litres each

Protein for growth and healing – in meat, fish, eggs, milk, cheese, yoghurt, nuts, beans and lentils, bread.

Carbohydrate for energy – in bread, flour, pasta, rice, cereals, sugar, fruit and vegetables.

Fats – in meat, fish, chicken, milk, cream, butter, oils, biscuits and cakes.

Calcium for strong bones and teeth – in milk, cheese and yoghurt, canned fish, green leafy vegetables, white bread.

Vitamin C to fight infection and aid healing – potatoes, citrus fruit such as oranges, fruit juice, green vegetables, berry fruits.

Some of the important food groups in a balanced diet.

day and a hot drink in cold weather is an essential part of your duties. Some people may need to have drinks (in a vacuum flask) and food left easily accessible to them. Supplement drinks that contain essential nutrients may often be prescribed and these should always be made according to the manufacturer's instructions. Being aware of clients' likes and dislikes and cultural dietary needs is also important. Always check that the meal is well presented and manageable especially if your client has difficulty chewing.

If a client has dentures you may want to ask them if these need cleaning or if they are well fitting and intact. Broken dentures can cause friction to the gums, contribute to oral infection and stop the person from eating altogether. Offer your client a bowl of water or help them to the bathroom to wash their hands before eating. Alternatively moist wipes may be used. If you are helping someone to eat by holding the cutlery, make sure that you are comfortable and relaxed. Make time so that you do not rush. Always check that the client will get a drink or food within a given time if you are not returning.

Helping clients to wash, dress and keep warm

The amount of help required by clients will vary according to their level of independence and ability. You may be required to help a client to take a bath or shower, to wash and dress at the sink or with a bowl or to give a bed bath.

The room should be warm, and it is important that you have towels and clean clothes ready to put on when the client has washed. Helping someone to wash also provides the opportunity to look for any skin rashes or breakdown of skin tissue and red areas that may lead to pressure sores. These should be recorded and reported to a qualified member of staff.

Always establish a trusting relationship so that the client feels able to perform very personal aspects of care in your presence. You can do this by ensuring that you know how you are going to help and what you are going to do, and encouraging them to tell you how they would like things done. Always remember to encourage clients to be involved in their own care and remember not to do anything that they can do for themselves, no matter how small.

If you feel that special equipment is needed such as a hoist or a bath seat, report this to a qualified member of staff. It will reduce the risk of any injury to you and may help your client to be more independent.

Dressing

Some clients will need help in both choosing clothes and dressing. Often clients depend upon other services to launder their clothes. Provide the client with a choice of what they want to wear and make sure that the clothes are appropriate to the temperature, and to the season. Ensuring that clients can manage zips and buttons is important in promoting independence and reducing frustration. Occupational therapists can perform specialist assessments and make practical suggestions to help.

Help with toileting

Discretion is of utmost importance when assisting clients with toileting, and you should respect the client's privacy at all times. By knowing in advance what the client needs you can help to make this aspect of care as dignified as possible.

A few examples include:
• helping a client to get out of bed/chair and walk to the toilet
• helping a client to transfer from a bed/chair to a commode
• helping a client to empty a colostomy bag
• helping a client manage incontinence.

You will need to know how to move clients safely when assisting with toileting. Always ensure that you have received adequate supervision for these tasks. This includes aspects of care such as emptying and observing a urinary catheter or changing a stoma bag.

A commode is often used in the bedroom and sometimes in the sitting room. Always try to imagine how you could feel in this situation. You can help to reduce embarrassment by ensuring that:

• all necessary equipment is gathered and the commode is clean and ready for use

• there is a clear space around the commode before you start

• doors and curtains are closed

• the commode is positioned in a way that will make the transfer easy for the client

• toilet tissue is at hand

• hand washing facilities are available

• the commode is emptied and returned to its original position

• if needed, air freshener is used discreetly.

Knowing the normal toilet habits and the words the client uses will help you to understand any difficulties experienced and know what to report to the trained nurse.

Always report the following:

• constipation

• blood in the stool

• incontinence of faeces or urine

• concentrated urine

• difficulties or pain in passing urine

• urine that smells "fishy"

• pink or blood stained urine

• urine testing results.

Mouth care

A clean and healthy mouth encourages appetite and prevents the mouth from being a focal point for infection. Clients may need help getting the necessary toiletries, with teeth cleaning, or with fitting or removing dentures. You should check to ensure that the client does not have any pain from damaged or infected teeth and that dentures fit properly. You should ask the client if they have a dry mouth, cracked lips, sores or ulcers. They may also tell you that they have a bad taste in their mouth. Clients who are dying can often be helped by simply giving regular sips of fluid to cleanse their mouth.

Eye care

All clients should be given help if required, to perform eye care and sometimes removal of eye make-up. Some clients may require eye care when eye drops are prescribed for a specific treatment. Always wash your hands before undertaking eye care for someone else. Cooled boiled water or a sachet of sterile saline and gauze or a tissue is preferable to cotton wool as small strands can break off into the eye. A different piece of gauze or tissue should be used to cleanse each eye to prevent infection being spread from one eye to the other. Some clients may have a false eye and need help with removing, cleaning and replacing the shell (you will be shown exactly how this is done).

Skin care and pressure areas

As someone who attends regularly to clients, you are in an ideal position to observe the condition of their skin. Always report red, sore, blistered or damaged skin. Skin care is especially important where clients may be incontinent of urine or faeces, where they spend time sitting or lying in one position and have difficulty moving about, and where clients may have poor nutrition and/or fluid intake.

Pressure sores arise because of poor blood supply to a part of the body caused by compression. This occurs where body tissues are squashed between a bone inside

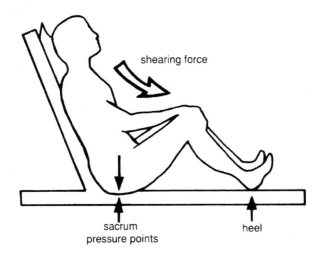

Fig 1. Pressure points.

the body and a firm surface such as a bed or chair. Susceptible areas include the buttocks, the heel of the foot, the hips and elbow joints.

Shearing and friction forces can also result in pressure sores. This occurs when a person is incorrectly lifted or allowed to slide down the bed or chair (Fig 1). The skin can become grazed and broken. Unless pressure is relieved, the skin tissue never has the opportunity to heal. Friction can also occur where one part of the body rubs against another, for example when a client in bed has one leg resting on another, or under the breasts.

Pressure relieving aids such as air cushions and mattresses, foam or sheepskins may be required to help patients who cannot easily move and relieve pressure themselves. There are many types of pressure relieving aids, although none will be as effective as actually moving the patient to relieve the site of pressure. You can help clients by reminding them of the need to change their position.

Besides observing your client's skin condition you may be asked to gently massage the pressure area to promote blood circulation. Moisturising creams can be applied to areas of unbroken dry skin or eczema as part of daily hygiene needs. In some circumstances a dressing may be applied to an area of broken skin to keep it dry and free from the risk of infection.

Wound care

A wound occurs where there is a loss of skin and this causes disruption to the normal tissue pattern. Wounds occur because of surgical operations, or injuries such as cuts, lacerations and tears. Wounds can also occur because of burns and chemical injuries and because of chronic ulceration due to poor blood supply or bacterial or viral infection.

Assessing a wound and selecting the correct product with which to treat it should always be undertaken by a qualified member of staff. The correct product will be dependent upon the type of wound, whether infection is present, the depth of the wound, the condition of the skin and any discharge. In addition the patient's general health and nutritional status will play a large part in successful wound healing. The most common wounds treated in the community include pressure sores and leg ulcers.

You are most likely to be asked to change a dressing where a client could normally perform this duty themselves, but because of illness or disability they are unable to do so.

The essential point of which you need to be aware is reducing the risk of cross infection. You should be taught how to replace a wound dressing using a non-touch or aseptic technique. Dressing Packs (sterile containers for dressing wounds) are designed so that you have minimum contact with any surface other than the wound cleanser, swabs and the dressing to be applied.

Always wash your hands before removing dressings and at the end of a procedure. Dispose of soiled dressings according to your local policy, usually in a sealable bag marked to show that it is clinical waste. Observe the wound and any changes to its condition. Replace the prescribed dressing as instructed by the qualified member of staff using a non-touch or aseptic technique.

Always record this activity when you have carried it out and report your findings to an appropriate team member. Take a note of the dressing packs or wound management products so that you can ensure that there will be an adequate supply for future treatments.

Encouraging and reinforcing advice to clients is just as important as changing a wound dressing. This may involve advising on position and movement, keeping limbs raised, ensuring a good diet and nutrition, promoting blood circulation by active movement, and preventing recurrence of the wound by avoiding knocks, or wearing special stockings or bandages.

Sexual health needs

Maintaining sexual health needs is about ensuring that each client can maintain their identity, perhaps by having the opportunity to dress as they would choose, to feel attractive, to have clean skin, clothes and so on. This may involve ensuring that your client can wear a perfume or aftershave of their choice, wear make-up or have their hair dressed.

Sexuality is also about relationships, a major part of each client's lifestyle. You may encounter relationships that are unlike your own, two men or two women who live and share their life together. Never judge other people's relationships, but respect their feelings, identity and lifestyle. They have the same right to respect, dignity and confidentiality as any other client. The way in which you communicate and react with people will have a direct bearing on the trust and confidence that they place in you at a time when they may be ill and most vulnerable. Your role in helping people to meet these basic human needs should never be underestimated.

Resting and sleeping

Adequate sleep or rest is important for people who are ill as the body needs time to rest and build up energy. All clients have different resting and sleeping patterns and you should be aware of these. It is important that you know what your client's usual sleeping habit and routines are. You may need to organise your visits to accommodate people who like to sleep late into the morning, nap in the afternoon or go to bed early or late. Always ask your clients how they have slept. Some may choose to sleep in a chair, particularly if they are in pain or have breathing problems.

Use pillows or back rests to position the client. Helping them to select warm clothing that does not restrict movement can enable them to be comfortable, move around and keep warm.

Advising and helping clients to use the

toilet before going to bed will prevent them being woken. A working bedside lamp or torch can be essential if people wake in the night and need to get up. It can also help people to feel more secure in the dark. The telephone or pendant alarm should also be within easy reach.

A commode near the bed may be less disruptive than having to struggle to a toilet, particularly if this is shared or outside the building. Sleeping medicines can also leave people feeling drowsy and unsteady on their feet. A commode may therefore be safer than travelling a long distance.

Slippers and shoes should be easily accessible and within reach at the bedside. A drink on the bedside table can save the client from having to get up. Check for draughts from open windows or under doors, and through floor boards.

Conclusion

Practical care is essential care. Promoting independence by providing essential care is paramount in enabling people with an illness or disability to maintain a good quality of life and to retain their dignity and privacy. An important point to remember is that you are a guest in your client's home. The first impressions you give to clients may make all the difference to having a good working relationship with them, and creating an atmosphere of trust.

Points to remember

1. Providing practical care will involve your contribution to assessing each individual client's needs.
2. Planning care needs to include the client, carer and other health, social service and independent agencies.
3. A care plan that is coordinated and agreed upon by all those involved will enhance client care.
4. Practical care and support is essential to many people who may live alone or to carers who need help.
5. Making clear and accurate records of any activity that you may carry out must be done as soon as possible.
6. Always report your observations or concerns to a qualified member of staff.

NVQ Levels 2 & 3 Core Units
O Promote equality for all individuals.
U4 Contribute to the health, safety and security of individuals and their environment.
U5 Obtain, transmit and store information relating to the delivery of of a care service.

Level 2 Core Units
Z1 Contribute to the protection of individuals from abuse.
W2 Contribute to the ongoing support of clients and others significant to them.
W3 Support clients in transition due to their care requirements.

Level 3 Core Units
Z8 Support clients when they are distressed.
Y2 Enable clients to make use of available services and information.

Level 2 Direct Care
Z6 Enable clients to maintain and improve their mobility.
Z7 Contribute to the movement and treatment of clients to maximise their physical comfort.
Z9 Enable clients to maintain their personal hygiene and appearance.
Z10 Enable clients to eat and drink.
Z11 Enable clients to access and use toilet facilities.
Z19 Enable clients to achieve physical comfort.

Level 2 Domiciliary Support
Z7 Contribute to the movement and treatment of clients to maximise their physical comfort.
Y1 Enable clients to maintain their domestic and personal resources.
W8 Enable clients to maintain contacts in potentially isolating situations.
U1 Contribute to the maintenance and management of domestic and personal resources.

CHAPTER 16

Caring for sick children at home

Alison Robertson

• Philosophy of care • Advantages of home care • The role of specialist paediatric care teams • Providing practical and emotional support • Practical care • Helping families and children with learning disabilities

Only a small proportion of all health and social care is delivered to children in hospital. Most of the care takes place at home, with the GP prescribing medication and treatment and parents or carers carrying out care with help from other agencies.

It is generally accepted that children should only be admitted to hospital when it is absolutely necessary and that children should stay in hospital only if they cannot be cared for at home, in the outpatient department or on a day care basis. Your role may involve providing care for sick children and their parents. Paediatric home care teams operate in many areas and provide specialist care for sick children at home.

Some children and their families require very short term care, such as single visits to replace dressings. Others have long term needs, such as those with cystic fibrosis, asthma, diabetes, cancer or because they have complex disabilities.

Philosophy of care

Children recover from accidents and illness more quickly in settings which are familiar to them and surrounded by those who love them. In order for this to take place some parents and carers may need help to cope with the worry of looking after a sick child. They may require teaching on how to undertake practical care and how to monitor progress and recovery.

Children may require referral to other specialist workers, such as child development teams who provide support, for example where children have a learning disability such as Down's Syndrome. Parents often require follow-up care and bereavement visiting if a child dies.

Advantages of home care

Caring for children at home can reduce the emotional trauma of an illness and promote recovery. It can avoid separation of the child from their family. It may be very costly for some families to make frequent visits to hospital. Travel and parking may be expensive or the hospital may be difficult to get to.

Keeping children at home can also reduce the risk of hospital-acquired infection. This can be very important if a child is suffering from an illness that makes them more susceptible to infection, such as leukaemia.

Caring for children at home enables the parent and the child to remain "in charge" of the situation. It also provides them with the opportunity to understand and learn about their illness. This enables them to contribute to their own care and recovery where possible and reduces disruption to their lives and normal development.

Paediatric home care teams

The role of specialist teams differs from area to area. Some provide care for children with specific conditions, others offer a general service to all children being treated by a specific hospital and GP. They are often designed to provide a service that is most suitable to the needs of the local population. This means that many teams adapt their service to accommodate special needs of the local population. An example could be multicultural health needs where sickle cell disease or thalassaemia (a condition affecting the blood) is more common.

It is useful to understand some specific roles of these specialist teams. This will help if you work directly with them. You may also receive specialist advice or support as part of your role in another team. The functions of the team usually include:

Direct practical care such as changing dressings, applying creams and lotions, giving medicines and drugs, helping with tube feeding and giving support and counselling.

Monitoring the child's condition. One way of avoiding hospital admission is to monitor the child's condition at home to assess the effects of any treatment that they may be receiving. Examples may

include physical examination such as regular weighing of the child, collecting specimens such as urine, taking regular recordings of pulse, temperature and blood pressure. Regular, planned visiting to monitor a child's condition at home can help to detect early signs of deterioration. This can prevent the condition from worsening and requiring hospital admission or unnecessary visits to the hospital outpatients department.

Educating the family and child. Teaching self-help programmes and enabling parents to care for their children is an important role of the paediatric home care team. Parents and children can be taught to carry out certain forms of treatment and care themselves. This enables them to be more independent and free to arrange their lives so that they can be as normal as possible.

Initially this can be quite a frightening experience for them. The correct technique, the reasons for carrying out the activity and regular reassurance are important to encourage these activities. Examples might include tube feeding or giving insulin injections for children with diabetes.

Coordinating and liaising with other services. A range of hospital, GP and other community services such as physiotherapists, child development teams, and speech therapists is available to help children and parents. Hospital admission can be avoided as home visits can be made. Treatment can be devised that fits in with the home environment and takes account of the needs of each family with least disruption.

Promoting early hospital discharge. By teaching parents and children how to undertake their own care it may be possible for discharge from hospital to take place much earlier. This has many advantages. Children can be reunited with their friends and playmates and perhaps attend school. It reduces the burden on parents who may wish to stay at the hospital but have other children or family members who depend on them. Discharge arrangements need to be in place before children leave hospital. This may mean visiting the child and family at the hospital to discuss the type and level of care and support needed. It may also mean making a home visit before discharge to make certain that everything required is in place. If specialist equipment is needed, or medicines and dressings, these need to be organised before the child leaves hospital.

Providing a choice of care. Some parents and carers lack the confidence to be able care for their child at home, even with support, and this option must be respected. Others however welcome the idea and feel happy at the prospect of looking after their child at home and establishing a more normal routine. Paediatric home care teams can increase the choice of treatment options available by advising parents of the range of choices and supporting them once they have made a choice.

Providing practical support. Each family must be carefully assessed and a decision agreed on the type and level of care that should be provided. As a health care assistant you can contribute to the assessment and planning of care. You may be required to participate in implementing, monitoring and reporting back any care activities that you carry out. It is essential that all members of the team are competent at teaching care to others. Most teams aim to work in partnership with family carers. This ensures that care of the child can be managed by the family

at the most appropriate time, when they feel able and confident.

Practical care

Outlined below are some common practical activities that you might be involved in. You should always make certain that you have been taught the correct procedure and that you feel confident and competent to carry it out. Always record the activities that you have carried out in the appropriate records and report back to a qualified member of staff.

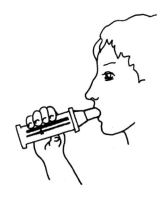

Fig 1. Using a peak flow meter.

Helping with breathing problems
Children can suffer from many problems with breathing, where the airways of the lungs become narrow and breathing becomes difficult. There are many causes. These include spasm and narrowing of the muscles around the airways in the lungs, inflammation of the lining of the airways, and swelling and excessive secretion of mucus. You may encounter children with asthma or cystic fibrosis. Although the cause and treatments are very different a common activity is to record the "Peak Flow" – how fast the person can blow out.

Peak flow meters (Fig 1) come in various forms. Each has a marker that moves out when a person blows into it.

The marker stops when the maximum speed of flow has been reached. The meter has a mouthpiece that the person blows into as hard and as quickly as they can. You must make certain that the mouth is sealed around the mouthpiece and that no air escapes. Three readings are usually taken, and the best one recorded.

Peak flow is usually measured on waking in the morning and in the evening. Readings can also be made before and after medicines.

Bronchodilators are medicines that can be inhaled directly into the lungs. They can be administered through inhalers or puffers. These are small hand-held machines, into which a tube of the medicine is inserted. A puff of the medicine is released as the person inhales air deeply into the lungs. Children can also benefit by taking inhalations through a nebuliser. This transforms liquid medications into a fine mist that is then breathed in through a mask.

Helping with eating problems
Enteral feeding is a system of providing vital nutrition. It may be used, for example, when the person is unable to chew or swallow but is still able to digest and absorb nutrients, or as a supplement to an insufficient diet. A tube can be passed via the nose or surgically into the stomach. Enteral feeds can be given at regular times during the day, or the tube feed can be connected to a pump and run continuously for several hours.

A qualified member of staff will usually be responsible for checking that the tube is correctly inserted before each feed, and that the site around the tube is not red, inflamed or swollen. If you are helping a qualified member of staff or parent you should ensure that you always wash your hands, and that all equipment is cleaned before and after administration.

The potential problems to look out for and report include nausea, vomiting and diarrhoea. The feed may be given too quickly or the strength may need to be adjusted by the dietician. Other problems that can occur include tube blockage. Feeds should always be prescribed by a dietician, stored safely and hygienically and given at room temperature.

Helping with skin problems
Body creams and lotions may need to be applied to children who have skin disease, such as eczema, or burns. Always wash your hands and wear disposable gloves to apply creams and lotions. This will prevent any chance of infection, particularly where the skin is broken.

If the skin needs to be cleaned before applying a new cream, check to ensure that you are using the appropriate cleanser. Soap and water may not always be the right choice, and sometimes other creams can be used to cleanse the skin before applying the medication.

Try to apply the cream or lotion as evenly as possible so that the correct penetration and absorption are achieved. Dressings may need to be applied to improve absorption and prevent the medicine from being accidentally rubbed off.

Helping with bone, joint and muscle problems
Traction, a system of stretching a limb, can be applied to children at home. This generally consists of weights attached to the body either surgically or with bandages, that hold it in a fixed position.

There are a number of reasons why this may be carried out. Examples include minimising muscle spasm or maintaining the correct position to correct a deformity or dislocation. Ensuring rest to a limb until healing has occurred and correcting or maintaining limb length where

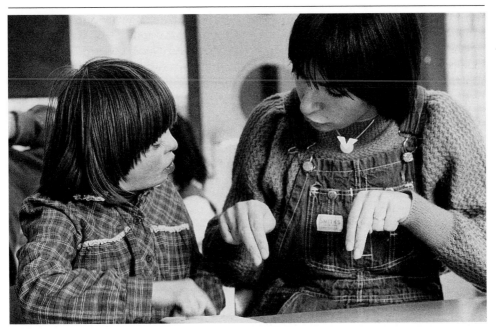

Children with disabilities may need greater stimulation than other children to achieve their potential.

shortening may have occurred due to disease or trauma, are other important examples.

The most important things to look out for include ensuring that the body and limbs are correctly aligned. This means ensuring that they are in the correct position to ensure successful traction and correct healing.

Pressure sores can occur, either where the body is forced to remain in one position or where the traction is applied to the body. Regular pressure relief and the use of special mattresses and aids such as air cushions and sheep skins can help to prevent this.

Boredom and lack of independence can be very frustrating to children, who may feel that the benefits of the traction are too long in coming, and not worth waiting for. Both parents and children can be helped to overcome this by suggesting regular and different forms of play and work activities.

Helping families and children with disabilities

Children can be born with physical and mental disabilities that can affect their ability to learn. Although medical intervention may be required, such as operations to correct deformities and medicines to prevent and treat illness, restoring the child to "normal" health is not always possible. Children with special needs can be helped to develop and achieve as normal a life as possible if they and their families receive special care, treatment and advice. Although children with a disability are not necessarily sick, they may be more susceptible to illness or require specialist help.

Child Development Teams are commonly available to help with children up to school leaving age. These teams are made up of doctors, nurses, psychologists, physiotherapists and occupational therapists.

To help the child to achieve their

potential they may need greater stimulation than other children. This may include helping them to play with toys that are appropriate to their abilities and encouraging them to concentrate on activities that they find difficult.

Some children who are unable to develop speech and language can be taught to use a type of sign language. This can help with communication and improve their ability to learn.

When the child reaches school age, the most appropriate type of education will be considered. Wherever possible, "special schools" are avoided and children are placed in mainstream schools so that they can continue to develop in as normal an environment as possible. You may need to support and listen to parents' anger, anxiety and frustrations. Ensuring that they know how to contact professionals when necessary can be just as important as carrying out practical care. Often, there are specialist support groups for parents of children with a learning disability. A knowledge of these agencies and encouraging membership and active participation can help parents to feel less isolated (see also Chapter 10).

Points to remember

1. Children should only be admitted to hospital when it is absolutely necessary.
2. Children recover from accidents and illness more quickly in settings which are familiar to them and surrounded by those who love them.
3. Caring for children at home enables the parent and the child to remain in charge of the situation and provides the opportunity for them to understand and learn about their illness.
4. Caring for children at home enables parents and children to contribute to care and recovery where possible and reduces disruption to their lives and normal development.
5. Paediatric home care teams can help children and their families by giving practical help and support; by monitoring a child's condition at home; by educating the child and family; by coordinating and liaising with other services; by promoting early hospital discharge and by ensuring a choice of care.

Further Reading
Baum D, Graham-Jones S (1991) *Child Health – The Complete Guide.* Penguin Books.

NVQ Level 2 & 3 Core Units
O Promote equality for all individuals.
U4 Contribute to the health, safety and security of individuals and their environment.
U5 Obtain, transmit and store information relating to the delivery of a care service.
Level 2 Core Unit
W2 Contribute to the ongoing support of clients and others significant to them.
Level 3 Core Units
Z8 Support clients when they are distressed.
Y2 Enable clients to make use of available services and information.
Level 2 Direct Care
Z6 Enable clients to maintain and improve their mobility
Z7 Contribute to the movement and treatment of clients to maximise their physical comfort.
Z9 Enable clients to maintain their personal hygiene and appearance.
Z10 Enable clients to eat and drink.
Z11 Enable clients to access and use toilet facilities.
Z19 Enable clients to achieve physical comfort.
Level 2 Domiciliary support
Z7 Contribute to the movement and treatment of clients to maximise their physical comfort.
W8 Enable clients to maintain contacts in potentially isolating situations.

CHAPTER 17

Lifting and handling clients

Stuart Darby

• How to assess the risk of lifting and handling a client • How to plan a lift
• Staff training • Methods of lifting • Recording and reporting risk factors

Moving furniture, carrying shopping and picking up children are just some of the everyday activities of lifting and handling that we take for granted. Lifting clients and supporting them to transfer from one position to another is an important part of the work of the care assistant. The danger of taking this type of activity for granted is that we no longer concentrate on what we are doing, and so increase the risks of injuring ourselves, our clients or work colleagues.

Important new regulations* came into force in January 1993. These regulations are designed to ensure that all people involved in manual lifting and handling are aware of these risks and only undertake lifting and handling when it is really necessary, as part of a conscious and planned decision.

The new lifting and handling regulations stress the importance for everyone involved in lifting to receive practical training in their place of work. This training should help you to contribute to assessing the risks involved in lifting and handling clients and to take account of your own abilities, the abilities of clients to help themselves, the

methods and equipment you may use and the surroundings in which you lift and handle. The regulations stress three main points:

• Lifting and handling should be avoided as far as reasonably practicable.

• Lifting should be planned by a suitably qualified member of staff, and these plans should be recorded and followed.

• Any identified risks or unsafe practices should be reported and recorded to prevent accidents or injury as a result of lifting and handling.

Assessing the risk

Before starting any lifting or handling procedure, the risks to both the client being lifted and the person undertaking the lift must be assessed so that steps can be taken to reduce any threat of injury. The key factors in assessment are:

1. The lifter's ability, knowledge, and fitness to lift.

2. The ability of the person being lifted to assist themselves.

3. The lifting and handling task to be undertaken.

125

4. The surroundings in which lifting and handling will take place.

5. Recording the lifting and handling method.

6. Steps to reduce or remove the risk of injury.

7. Lifting and handling methods.

These key factors are considered in detail in this chapter.

1 The lifter's ability, knowledge, and fitness to lift.

Training and education

Any person required to lift and handle must be offered the opportunity to participate in training and education tailored to their individual needs and the place in which they work.

Training should be provided by qualified practitioners and should aim to provide you with instruction, experience and a knowledge of:

• The Health & Safety at Work Act 1974 and the legal aspects of lifting and handling.
• How the body works in relation to movement and lifting and handling.
• How to assess any risks of injury and report to managers
• How to plan the most appropriate methods for safer client handling.
• Manual handling techniques and the use of equipment.
• Warning of unsafe handling practice.

Fitness to do the job

It is also important to ensure that as a lifter you are fit to undertake these duties. If you are not fit, you are at risk of back injury because of the strenuous nature of the job. Good health can contribute to your ability to make a reasoned assessment and your proficiency in undertaking the lift.

More than a quarter of accidents at work reported each year are associated with manual handling. The majority result in injuries lasting over three days and occur because of prolonged lifting over a period of time rather than as a result of single accidents. These injuries can result in long term physical problems or even permanent disability.

Appropriate clothing and footwear

Uniforms should be designed to take into account the movements that you will need to make. They must allow you to bend and stretch freely. Where no uniform is worn, it is important that you select clothing that allows free movement, but is unlikely to be caught in equipment. Footwear, in particular rubber soled shoes, will protect you from static electricity and are non-slip on wet or polished surfaces. The upper surface is equally important to protect feet from articles or objects that may be dropped on them.

2 The ability of the person to assist themselves

Promoting independence

Apart from reducing the risk of injury to lifters, promoting independence is important because it allows each person the opportunity to assist and control everyday tasks, to do what they want to, when they need to. It allows each person to have a sense of dignity and fulfilment in carrying out movement and daily living activities without interference and intrusion.

There are however a number of physical and psychological factors that need to be considered in assessment that will prevent or limit the extent to which some clients can assist themselves in lifting and handling. In order to plan the best approach you should also refer to other chapters in this book.

Factors affecting clients' ability to assist with lifting and handling include:

Physical factors.

• The weight, height and shape of the person.

• Normal "wear and tear" to the body, or the process of an illness or disease.

• Decreased elasticity of muscles and the inability to bend and flex easily.

• A decline in strength of bones through bone loss.

• Reduced lung expansion causing breathlessness on effort.

• Poor eyesight and inability to recognise objects, steps or floor changes increases the risk of falls and accidents.

• Changes in the inner ear may cause loss of balance control.

• Medicines and alcohol causing drowsiness and unsteadiness.

• Heart changes, causing blood pressure to rise or fall quickly, may make the person dizzy or unsteady.

• Pain in the hands or limbs, caused through rheumatism or arthritis, can limit a full range of movement.

• The effects of tiredness.

• Other physical constraints (drips, tubes, splints, traction).

Psychological factors

• The ability to remember and recall information or to recognise places or objects, where they are (the time, month or year), and what is happening to them.

• The ability to communicate, speak or to understand what is being said.

• The ability to behave appropriately, including aggression due to frustration, confusion, anxiety or suspicion of any actions carried out.

• "Clinging", which can occur where the person has experienced a fall, feels insecure and has lost self confidence.

• Understanding of the situation (which may be impaired where there has been damage or disease of the brain).

• The mood of the person (happy and relaxed or sad and anxious) may affect their ability to concentrate, or their willingness and motivation to participate.

3 *The lifting and handling task to be undertaken*

Do I need to lift and handle?
The first question before any lifting task is whether it actually needs to be undertaken, or whether the person can move themselves.

Where lifting or assistance is needed, the point at which the lift will start from and where it will end needs to be clarified. If you are required to twist, stretch or bend in order to carry out the task there is an added risk of injury. The length of time that the lift takes will add to the risk of injury, particularly if it is to be repeated on several occasions during the day. The plan for repeated and regular lifting therefore, needs to ensure that the least stress is placed upon the person and the lifters.

What method should be used?
The type of lifting carried out will depend upon the assessment and characteristics of the person to be lifted, your own abilities, the environment in which you will lift and handle and the range of equipment and staff available to help you.

Preparation for the type of lift to be carried out
The following checklist is a guide to selecting which method of lift to use:

• Can this lift be undertaken manually or does equipment need to be used ?

• Is it a horizontal transfer lift? Can a sliding action be used?

• Does the lift involve pivoting or turning?

• Is it a vertical lift? How much weight has to be lifted?

• Does it involve turning the person in bed?

• What level of support does the person need?

• Is there an additional task to be done, eg changing clothes or using a bedpan?

• Will you be able to maintain a good posture, keeping your body symmetrical and your back straight?

• Do you need more staff to help?

• What equipment may be needed?

Hoists

Hoists may be used for lifting clients in or out of bed, for lifting a person up the bed, raising a person while the lower sheets are changed or the person is being washed, and for lifting clients in the bath and from the floor.

Hoists may be fixed in a certain place, such as bathrooms or they may be mobile. If they are mobile it is essential that you always remember to apply the brakes. Hoists also have many attachments such as seat fittings and slings. You should always use the correct fitting. Remember that there are always manufacturers' representatives who will advise and can even have specially adapted slings made.

Handling or transfer equipment

Equipment is designed to be used as an aid to lifters. Handling and transfer equipment is also designed to be used by clients who can assist themselves and so increase their level of independence after being taught how to use it safely. Practical examples are included in *Lifting and handling methods* below.

All equipment needs to be selected with care, regularly inspected for wear and tear and regularly maintained. If it is available it should always be used. Advice on equipment can be sought from qualified staff, physiotherapists, occupational therapists, or the manufacturers of the equipment. Always seek special training in the use of mechanical hoists.

4 The surroundings in which the lift is taking place

Is the area clear ?

Ensure that you have enough space in which to move around, and that the distance you will be travelling is clear of any objects or items of furniture. If you are transferring a person from one place to another, for example bed to chair, ensure that these are at the same level.

Plan your move to take into account the number of different stages, standing, turning, sitting and so on. Lower any handrails or chair sides to minimise the amount of lifting and lowering required. Be sure to lock the wheels of equipment, and position, for example, a chair or bed ladder which may help the client to help themselves.

If you are involved in lifting at night, make sure that the area is well lit and that you can see where you are going.

Is the floor safe?

There may be obstacles, such as furniture or rugs and carpets. The floor may be wet, polished or may be covered in talcum powder, or other slippery substances. Do remember that other people and/or pets may be a hazard to look out for.

Clothing and footwear of the person be lifted

It is equally important, where appropriate, for the person being lifted and handled to wear well fitting shoes that support the foot and ankle, and not loose fitting slippers. Remember also that long hair, rings and jewelry can get trapped in clothing and equipment.

5 Recording the lifting and handling method

Care planning

It is good practice for a trained "assessor" to be responsible for making an initial assessment and for documenting care needs in partnership with the client. A trained assessor is usually a qualified nurse or therapist who has undertaken specialist education in assessing lifting and handling risks and identifying the most appropriate methods and equipment to be used. Assessors are responsible for written care plans and nursing records. Re-assessment should take place whenever required, and following regular review.

Written plans for lifting and handling should include:

- The lift to be carried out.
- How the lift will be carried out.
- The number of lifters required.
- Any environmental considerations or precautions to be taken
- The type of equipment required.
- Agreement that everyone involved, including the person to be lifted, understands the methods to be used and how they might help.

The specific responsibility for each handling task however, lies with each lifter on every occasion that a lift is undertaken. You are responsible for reading and following the care plan. Changes in care should be reported and care plans altered as soon as possible. Where difficulties exist these must be recorded and reported as soon as possible.

6 Steps to reduce or remove the risk of injury

Employer responsibilities

Your employer has a responsibility to ensure that you are fit to lift and handle by providing training, a safe environment and by ensuring that you have the appropriate equipment where available. As an employee you also have a responsibility for the safety of yourself, the clients that you are lifting and

handling and the other staff with whom you work. This includes reporting injuries and where there is a lack of resources and equipment.

Injuries, accidents or illness at work

Your manager has a responsibility to ensure that neither the person you are lifting, yourself or your colleagues are exposed to a foreseeable risk of injury from lifting and handling.

Your responsibility is to aim to reduce the risk of injury by reporting and recording where there is a problem or where work place injuries or accidents have occurred. This includes any illness or disability affecting your handling abilities when you are new to post or in the course of your duties, whether relating to a work accident or not. This can be done confidentially through occupational health services and GPs.

Reducing and removing the risk of injury

In order to reduce and remove the chance of injury it is good practice to record and report any risks to your manager. This includes the following:

a) Lack of staff or equipment.
b) Environmental hazards.
c) Defects in machinery or equipment.
d) Injuries or accidents.
e) Any illness or disability affecting your handling ability.

a) Lack of staff or equipment.

- What type of equipment is needed and why?
- Why are more staff required on this occasion?
- Has any previous action been taken?

b) Environmental hazards

- Where does the environmental hazard exist?
- What is the environmental hazard creating difficulty?
- What immediate action can remove or reduce the hazard?

c) Defects in equipment/machinery used for lifting
- What model of equipment is it?
- Has it been maintained recently?
- What is the defect or problem?

d) Injuries or accidents
- When and how did the injury occur?
- What equipment was involved?
- What medical treatment was given or action taken?

e) Any illness or disability affecting your handling ability
- How does this limit your ability to lift and handle?
- Do you need to take any special precautions?
- Do you need any special equipment, or have other requirements?

7 Lifting and handling methods

Holds and lifts
The following limited holds and lifts are intended to illustrate the need for safe and planned lifting and handling. The risks associated with lifting and handling are complex. No responsibility can be accepted for any decisions made solely upon the information in this chapter.

Each individual has a responsibility to ensure that they are trained and competent, are able to assess situations to the best of their abilities and have had the opportunity to participate in demonstrations and controlled practice with a qualified practitioner.

It is essential that explanation of the lift is given to the client and that the lifter gains cooperation where possible.

HOLDS AND LIFTS: ONE HANDLER
These holds are intended to support and move the person who is able to give some assistance and to bear some of their own weight. They are used to assist a person to stand or transfer from one seated

position to another seated position close by – for example from wheelchair to toilet.

For the following holds it is essential that the person is sitting well towards the front of the chair or bed, leaning forward and bringing their centre of gravity over their feet which are well tucked in.

- Handling belt hold (Figure 1)
- The lifting block (Figure 2)
- The turn-table (Figure 3)
- Through arm grasps (Figure 4)

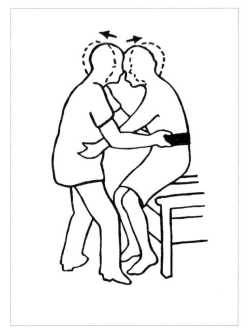

Figure 1: Handling belt hold (above)

1) Stand in front and to one side of the sitting person.

2) Place one foot beside them and the other in front – blocking the person's knees.

3. Insert thumbs in a wide belt (at least three inches) that is secured around the person and grasped. Special belts are available for this purpose.

4. Ask the person to support themself by pushing up on the arms of a chair or by putting their hands on the lifter's hips.

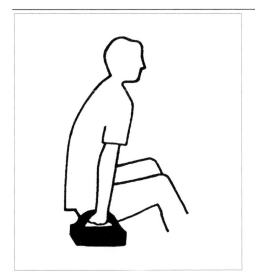

Figure 2: The lifting block (above)

This is useful for patients who may have limited power on one side of the body only.

1) As the lifter lifts, the person pushes down onto the block from a slightly bent elbow on the strong side of the body and pushes onto the strong heel.

2) The lifter adopts the position for the shoulder lift (Figure 8) on the person's weak side but the palm is placed upwards under the person's near thigh, at the same time locking the person's arm if it is paralysed.

Figure 3: The turntable (right)

This may be used for selected clients with caution. It is not suitable for people who are confused or cannot be relied upon to take weight through their knees.

1) Place the person's feet firmly on the turntable and stand to one side of them

2) Hold them with the axillary hold, or belt and keeping close to their body, help them to stand

3) The lifter pushes the turn-table round with their foot until the person is in the correct position to sit on the chair or edge of the bed provided.

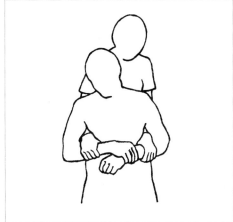

Figure 4: Through arm grasp (above)

1) Hold the person's forearm close to their body. Their stronger hand should grasp the weaker wrist (if appropriate).

2) Stand directly behind them.

3) Grasp as near to their wrist as possible, and tuck their hands into the lower abdomen

This lift is used where the person is seated in an upright position and where they are able to stand, carry some of their own weight, understand and cooperate.

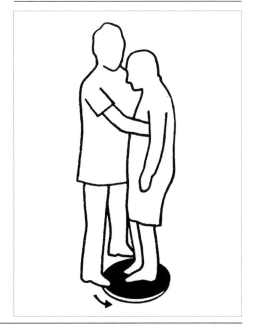

HOLDS AND LIFTS: TWO HANDLERS

Two handlers sharing a lift will still in effect be each bearing two thirds of the total load. The weight may also be unevenly distributed – for example when one lifter has the shoulders and trunk and a second lifter has the feet. At least two lifters should be used where they are manually lifting the whole weight of a person.

- Handling sling (Figure 5)
- Double wrist (Figure 6)
- Double forearm (Figure 7)

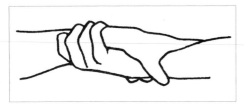

Figure 5: Handling sling (above)

The handling sling should be used in order to extend the reach and reduce a stooping or twisting action. In the absence of a sling a double wrist hold or a finger hold should be used.

1) The handling sling is placed high up under the person's thighs and the lifters hold the sling instead of each others hands.

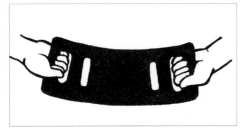

Figure 6: Double wrist hold (above)

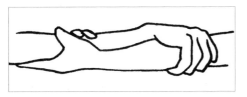

Figure 7: Double forearm hold (above)

Moving clients in bed

- The shoulder lift (Figure 8)
- The through arm lift – up the bed (Figure 9)

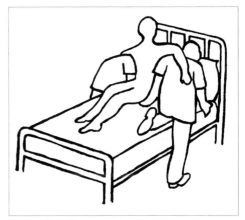

Figure 8: The shoulder lift (above)

Moving in bed or transferring to a chair

1) Adjust the bed to a height halfway between your hips and knees.

2) Apply the brakes

3) Lifters stand on opposite sides to each other with their feet apart.

4) The leading foot should face the moving direction.

5) The hips and knees are bent, with the back straight.

6) Lifters press their near-side shoulders into the chest wall under the person's arms as shown, while the client rests their hands and arms down your backs.

7) Grip your partner using the wrist grip.

8) Place your hands on the bed behind the client to support their trunk, with elbows flexed ready to take the weight.

9) Leading lifter gives the command "lift".

10) Slowly straighten your trailing legs and elbows.

11) Lift clear of the bed and then lower by bending the leading legs and supporting elbows.

12) Only move the client for a short distance at a time.

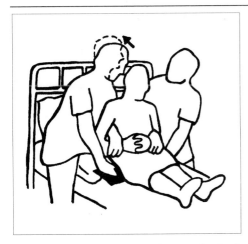

Figure 9: Through arm lift - up the bed or into a chair (above)

1) Put your knee on the bed behind the client.

2) Using the "through arm grasp", move them to the side of the bed.

3) Place your feet on the floor, behind the client, while continuing to support them.

4) Second lifter positions the chair, then faces the bed with their feet one in front of the other.

5) Second lifter slides their hands under the person's legs.

6) On command, the second lifter pulls the person's legs to the side of the bed, and supports their weight.

7) Lift (using the through arm grasp).

8) Move in this way, for the shortest distance possible, and gently lower to the chair.

Turning the person in bed

Lifting is unnecessary when turning a person in bed. Turning involves rolling and sliding TOWARDS the lifter. This can be achieved in a number of ways.

• Draw sheet or polythene sheet

• Handling sling

• Easy-glide boards (Figure 10)

Draw sheet and polythene sheet

A draw sheet or strong sheepskin placed over a polythene sheet to ease gliding can be used to pull the person into position. They should always be supported and comfortable. Care should be take to avoid any friction to the person's skin. No reaching movements should be made away from the lifter, only towards the lifter.

Handling slings

Two handling slings can be used where there is no draw-sheet. These are positioned under the person's thighs and lower back. Feet, head and shoulders are moved first and then lifters on either side of the bed hold the slings to pull and roll the person's pelvis and trunk.

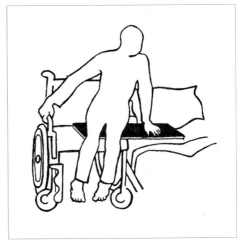

Figure 10: Easy glide board (above)

Easy glide boards are designed to be placed under the person. Specific practical instruction is required to ensure safe use of this equipment.

The falling or fallen client

Teaching people to fall and rise safely is a skilled activity. Training should be provided by qualified practitioners and should aim to provide the handler and the client with instructions and practical experience.

Clients who are at risk of falling should be taught firstly, how to fall safely and then how they should rise.

Lifting clients who have fallen to the floor is a very high risk activity. The first task is to ensure that the client is reassured and made comfortable. Check that they have not sustained any injury. Help should always be summoned and an assessment and well organised lift, preferably using a mechanical hoist, is essential.

Points to remember

1. Each individual has a responsibility to ensure that they are trained, competent, and able to assess situations to the best of their abilities.
2. Never lift a person unless you have to; always consider alternatives.
3. Ensure that everyone involved, including the person you are lifting, knows and understands the plan of lifting and handling: what each person is expected to do, what equipment will be used and any special precautions that need to be taken.
4. Never undertake a lift where the individuals cannot be held close to the body or if your back is twisted.
5. Make certain that there is enough space to lift, it is well lit and that there are no obstacles such as furniture, or hazards such as a slippery floor.
6. Always seek help to move another person unless you are absolutely certain they require minimal support.
7. Never try to stop a person falling – guide them to the floor.

8. Never lift a person out of the bath or from the floor – use a hoist or bath seat.
9. Never hold the weight of a client while a nursing activity is being carried out such as wound care or changing clothing or bed linen.
10. Always report to the appropriate manager where there are insufficient staff or equipment, an unsafe environment or faulty equipment with which to lift and handle.

Further reading

*EEC (1990) *Minimum Health and Safety requirements for handling loads where there is a risk of back injury for workers*. Directive 90/269. EEC.

The Guide to the Handling of Patients 3rd Ed. National Back Pain Association in Collaboration with the Royal College of Nursing (1992).

NVQ Levels 2 & 3 Core Units
O Promote equality for all individuals.
U4 Contribute to the health, safety and security of individuals and their care environment.
U5 Obtain, transmit and store information relating to the delivery of a care service.
Level 2 Core Unit
W2 Contribute to the ongoing support of clients and others significant to them.
Level 3 Core Unit
Y2 Enable clients to make use of available services and information.
Level 2 Direct Care
Z6 Enable clients to maintain and improve their mobility.
Z7 Contribute to the movement and treatment of clients to maximise their physical comfort.
Z9 Enable clients to maintain their personal hygiene and appearance.
Level 2 Domiciliary Support
Z7 Contribute to the movement and treatment of clients to maximise their physical comfort.

CHAPTER 18

Promoting continence and stoma care

Helen White and Stuart Darby

• How we all feel about bladder and bowel control • Passing urine • How the bowel works
• What is continence and how is it achieved? • Problems that can lead to incontinence
• Assessing the type of incontinence • Incontinence of faeces • Toileting programmes
• Personal protection • Catheter care and hygiene • Sex • Stoma care

Going to the lavatory is a basic human activity which we all perform several times a day without much thought and rarely discuss unless something goes wrong.

Our culture seems to find it hard to cope with anything to do with bladders and bowels: the public are embarrassed by the subject, many professionals tend to ignore the problems, and too often care assistants are simply left to cope as best they can.

This chapter will discuss how clients and care staff feel about this sensitive and intimate part of care; explain how continence is achieved and maintained; describe what may go wrong, how incontinence can be managed, and what resources are available.

Confusing terms

Continence is not an easy subject to talk about. It is hard to find words that are descriptive and easy to use, so we often use euphemisms such as "relieving yourself", but these terms can also cause confusion and embarrassment. Nurses and doctors resort to clinical terms which are little understood by most people.

Feelings

Incontinence can have devastating effects, especially when symptoms are obvious such as wet chairs and smelly clothes. Some people will go to extraordinary lengths to hide their incontinence, either denying there is a problem and refusing to seek help, or isolating themselves from families and friends. Feelings of shame, helplessness, rejection and misery are commonly expressed.

It is generally assumed that care staff are at ease with all aspects of toileting and incontinence, but we can be just as embarrassed as anyone else at having to assist clients perform these intimate tasks. We too can feel disgusted that someone is not able to control their bladder or bowel, and be resentful that we have to deal with the mess and the smell.

It is important to recognise and be aware of these feelings in ourselves, and

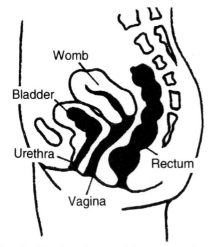

Female side view shows pelvic floor and body passages.

They act as a filter and remove waste products from the blood. These, in the form of urine, pass down two tubes, ureters, into the bladder. The bladder is an "elastic" bag made of muscle which expands to store the urine and contracts to squeeze the urine out through a narrow tube, the urethra, which is 4cm long in women, 20cm in men. The bladder and urethra are supported in position by the pelvic floor muscles.

When the bladder fills to about 250-350mls, it sends messages to the nerves in the lower part of the spine. These messages travel up the spine to the brain. The brain responds by sending the appropriate message back to the bladder. If the time and place are convenient, the nerves send the messages back down the spine to the bladder muscles. The bladder muscles contract, the urethra relaxes and the urine is squeezed out.

If the time and place are not convenient it is possible to ignore the desire to pass urine, and it will fade from consciousness. Then it returns at intervals until the need is so urgent that emptying can no longer be delayed.

to be able to share them with other staff, because in our care work we must always put ourselves in the client's place and imagine how *they* feel. You need to be very sensitive and discreet, especially when a client is denying that a problem exists. People have been ostracised and humiliated because of their incontinence: this is always totally unacceptable.

Incontinence can happen at all ages: children who wet the bed, young women who leak when they sneeze and men anxious about their prostate problems.

Everyone has an important part to play in the promotion of continence: as a care assistant you are closest to the client, the person they confide in, the one who performs the most intimate tasks. Talking to clients with knowledge and confidence will give them the reassurance that they are not alone and the guidance to where help is available.

Passing urine

Urine is produced in the kidneys. There are two kidneys situated in the lower part of the back on either side of the spine.

How the bowel works

In normal bowel action, the formed stool is pushed into the lower part of the bowel, called the rectum, by contraction of the muscular walls of the bowel. This triggers sensory receptors in the wall of the rectum which are felt as a desire to empty the bowel. The ring of muscle controlling the anus (the back passage outlet) is relaxed if the time and place is convenient, and the stool is passed, sometimes with the assistance of the muscles of the abdomen.

In a normal bowel action the stool is soft, well formed and easy to pass. Little hard pellets can indicate constipation.

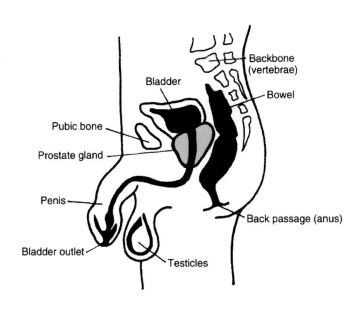

Side view of male showing enlarged prostate gland.

What is continence?

Continence is being able to pass urine or faeces voluntarily in a socially acceptable place. That is: recognising the need to go; holding on until it is convenient and comfortable; identifying the correct place; then emptying the bladder or bowel completely.

This requires a urinary and bowel system which is working effectively; a nervous system which can convey messages; the ability to move independently or at will, and toilet facilities which are easy to reach and acceptable.

Successful toilet training requires normal physical development, especially of the nervous system, and certain social skills such as being able to remove and replace clothing as necessary at the lavatory; being able to get up and walk to the lavatory, or ask to be taken, or ask for the lavatory; and being able to plan ahead for the lavatory whether the bladder is full or not.

Going to the lavatory demands a complex sequence of events:

• recognising the need to empty the bladder or bowel – so there must be no interruption in the nerve pathway between the bladder and the control centre in the brain

• holding on until an appropriate place is reached, even if the bladder is full (this can be particularly difficult for dependent clients who may have to wait for a helper)

• adjusting clothing – undoing zips, pulling down trousers

• sitting or standing at the lavatory, initiating the urine stream (or bowel movement) and sustaining it until the bladder or bowel is empty

• wiping the bottom or shaking the penis (it is very important for little girls to be taught to wipe from front to back to avoid the risk of infection)

• flushing the lavatory and making sure it is clean (no urine dribbles on the seat or soiling on the bowl)

• replacing clothes correctly and washing hands before leaving the bathroom.

It is also a very exhausting activity for people who have walking and handling difficulties or tire easily, and for clients with heart problems, arthritis or multiple sclerosis.

At what age is continence achieved?

Continence is seen as a major milestone of normal child development. All babies automatically empty their bladder and bowel when they are full, as a reflex action. The age of achieving control varies according to the child's physical and social development and cultural background. The accepted sequence is bowel control by night followed by bowel control by day; bladder control by day followed by bladder control at night.

At two years 50 per cent of children will have acquired bowel control and most will have bladder control during the day by three years and night control by four years. At around 18 months there is an awareness of the bladder and a brief holding of urine, and at three years a holding on for longer periods with an increasing bladder capacity. Between the ages of three and four the child should be able to initiate the stream when sitting on the lavatory, and by six years should be able to voluntarily start a stream without a full bladder. Girls generally acquire control before boys.

What are the problems?

The following questions will highlight the physical, emotional and environmental factors essential to maintaining continence:

Can they recognise the need to go?
Children with spina bifida and adults who are confused may not get the message and there are occasions when both they and others need reminding, for instance little boys holding on to their penis, or older people who are becoming restless. This will be discussed further under toileting programmes.

Can they ask to go?
Young children may use family words such as "poo-poo" to express their need to go to the toilet. Adults who have lost their speech following a stroke may have a special way of communicating; clients who have severe learning difficulties may communicate in a sign language. It is always advisable to check with family or friends to save embarrassment and distress.

Do they know where the lavatory facilities are?
Clear directions which are reinforced with signs will assist clients in their independence. Signs can also be used in a person's home if they are confused or forgetful. Some clients may prefer or find it easier to use a commode or urine bottle. Whenever possible encourage them to sit on the lavatory or commode as this is less stressful and more efficient than a bedpan. With guidance, each individual should make their own choice. Remember to give instructions on how to use urine bottles. Although they are familiar to you, many people will not-know what to do and may be too embarrassed to ask.

Can they get there in time?
The toilet should be within easy reach. If your client has walking problems and is slow it may be important that their bed or chair is as close to the door as possible. Shoes and a walking aid may help. If despite all this they don't get there in time, it is better to wheel them to the lavatory if necessary, and allow them to walk back slowly rather than suffer the humiliation of wetting on the way.

Care should be taken to ensure that the entrances to the toilet are free from obstruction and not used as an extra storage place, causing added delay.

Can they manage their clothing?
Easy-to-adjust clothing, such as an extended fly with dabs of velcro on trousers and

pyjamas, will overcome the difficulty for men of getting the penis out quickly enough, and women may find a fuller skirt where the back can be tucked into the belt, and split-crotch or French knickers quicker if there are problems with handling. Shoes give more support than slippers for easier walking.

Is the lavatory seat at an appropriate height?
The correct position is to sit with the bottom and back well supported and feet firmly on the ground. Little girls can be particularly scared about falling into the bowl, and many people crouch so as not to touch the seat for fear of infection.

In some cultures it is customary to squat with the feet on the seat. Do make sure that the seat and any surrounding rails are secure and able to take this unusual distribution of weight.

Clients who have difficulties balancing, or getting on and off the lavatory, will find aids such as grab rails helpful. The occupational therapist will advise on the positioning of the rails. Clients who need to push themselves up off the loo will require horizontal rails, while those who pull themselves up will need a vertical rail. A foot rest, and if necessary straps to support the trunk, give extra security and confidence. A raised seat is helpful for clients with stiff joints, and men with prostate problems may find sitting a more effective way of emptying their bladder.

Is the lavatory acceptable and private?
Finding a public lavatory quickly and easily can be one of the problems encountered by people with incontinence problems. Clients may feel at greater ease if they know where the nearest clean, well lit, warm and ventilated lavatory, with a door that locks, is available.

Trying to pass water and even worse having a bowel movement, when you are aware someone can hear and smell you, is most inhibiting. These problems can be overcome by running water, lining the pan with paper and spraying with a deodoriser.

Is cleaning adequate?
Clients who are soiled through faecal incontinence should be cleaned as soon as possible, using large soft tissues or special wipes, then washed with warm water and dried thoroughly. If the soiling has dried on to the skin, cleansing agents which can be sprayed on to the skin and then wiped off with a moist tissue are very helpful, particularly where the skin is already fragile.

Urine is acidic and can cause skin soreness, which in turn can lead to rashes and infection. Avoid scented soap and talcum powder as these can add to the irritation. A flannel for washing face and hands should be kept separately from the one used for washing between the legs. If the skin is particularly sensitive, patting between the legs with a soft towel or drying with a cool hairdryer can be helpful. A qualified member of staff staff will advise you on skin and barrier creams.

People from certain cultures, such as Moslems and Sikhs, hold strong views about personal hygiene, and may for example require a special jug so they can wash with running water. If in doubt it is best to ask family or friends.

How much are they drinking?
Many people believe they should drink less so that less urine will be passed. What happens, though, is that the urine becomes concentrated, the bladder capacity may become smaller and other problems can result, including constipation. A good guide is six cups of fluid for children and 10 cups for adults over 24 hours. Do encourage more water and less tea, coffee and cola, as these drinks stim-

ulate the kidneys to produce more urine than necessary.

Parents often teach their children to go to the lavatory each time they go to the shops, school or a journey. This habit of going at every opportunity trains the bladder to empty before it is full, and it often persists throughout adulthood so these people will never venture far from a public toilet. Anyone who requires to pass urine more than every two hours or who gets up more than twice a night, unless they are on medication, requires investigation.

Bowel frequency is very individual – once a day, twice a week – what is important is the *consistency*, not frequency. Stools should be soft, formed and easy to pass; straining to pass a stool can indicate constipation.

Certain medicines, such as water tablets (diuretics) increase the amount of urine, sometimes very rapidly, so the indivdual is given little warning. Sleeping tablets (sedatives) can delay the message being relayed and responded to by the brain; pain killers (analgesics) can cause constipation.

What is their attitude to continence?
Anxiety may cause both children and adults to wet themselves in a stressful situation. This may be acceptable for the child, but not for the older person. Such a humiliating experience is a memory which will never fade.

Depression can affect anyone – children as well as older people, and may lead to a loss of motivation. This should not be confused with laziness and attention-seeking. Loss of independence can lead some clients to use bladder and bowel control to their advantage; for many it is the only means they have left to express themselves. Forcing clients to the lavatory can have the opposite effect to the one you want.

Incontinence

Incontinence means the uncontrolled (involuntary) loss of urine or faeces. It is not a disease but a symptom of an underlying problem which can happen to anyone at any time of life. It affects more women than men but it is not an inevitable consequence of old age or disability. Indeed the majority of people remain continent all their lives.

Incontinence at any age causes physical, emotional, social and financial hardship and severely disrupts people's lives. Many see incontinence in older people as a natural stage of regression to infancy and treat them accordingly, increasing dependence and loss of adult status.

There are many causes of incontinence and an individual can suffer from several symptoms. Treatment or management must be based on individual assessment and investigation to discover the type of incontinence and possible causes.

Assessment

Assessment is based on answers to questions such as the following:

Do you leak when you cough or sneeze?
Leaking of urine on exertion, **stress incontinence**, can occur when there is extra strain on the tummy, such as coughing or sneezing. It is a common complaint in women of all ages, who have weakened muscles around the bladder and urethra during pregnancy and childbirth, after the menopause and if there is a history of constipation.

It can be cured by exercises to strengthen these muscles, and in extreme cases by surgery to tighten the muscles. It can be successfully managed by not letting the bladder become over-full, avoiding constipation, doing pelvic floor exercises, and wearing protective garments.

Do you have to go frequently and quickly?

A strong need to pass urine quickly and often, sometimes not reaching the lavatory in time because the bladder muscles become overactive and contract with little warning, is known as **urge incontinence.** The person rushes to the lavatory immediately they are aware of their bladder in an effort to prevent urine loss. The bladder seldom holds more than a few millilitres of urine because it is emptied so frequently. This quickly becomes a habit, and the time between emptyings becomes less and less – in extreme cases every 15 minutes.

It is common to men and women, particularly those who have problems affecting the nervous system, such as multiple sclerosis or stroke, those with dementia, and children and adults who are bedwetters. Sometimes people become so depressed and anxious about having an accident that they refuse to be far from a lavatory.

This type of incontinence is particularly common in older people. Again it is curable in many cases, by introducing a programme of bladder exercises to extend the intervals between trips to the lavatory, and wearing light protective garments to gain confidence. Medicines to quieten the bladder muscles may also be prescribed.

Do you have to get up at night?

Dribbling or continuous leakage of urine, sometimes leading to wetting the bed at night, is known as **overflow incontinence**. It is often associated with an obstruction at the bladder neck, such as an enlarged prostate gland (in men) or constipation. It may be due to the bladder muscles not contracting properly, for example where there is damage to the nerves of the spinal chord, so the bladder does not empty completely, retaining a substantial volume of urine which causes a feeling of fullness even after urine has been passed.

If left untreated this can lead to repeated urinary infections and other serious complications, so a medical assessment is important. How the condition is managed will depend on the cause, but always check for constipation and provide personal and bed protection to preserve the client's comfort and dignity. In some cases an intermittent or indwelling catheter (see page 144) will be recommended.

Do you find you get no warning?

The bladder may empty without any warning – **reflex incontinence** – because the nervous system is not conveying the messages to the brain. This may happen following spinal injury, extreme confusion or fear, or in children following an accident or acute illness.

In some cases a chart recording the times of the reflex can indicate a pattern which will allow toileting at set intervals to anticipate the loss, or it may be necessary for the urine to be contained with highly absorbent pads or another recommended method.

Can you get there in time?

Simply not getting to the lavatory in time because of walking and handling difficulties – **functional incontinence** – can usually be managed with easy-to-wear clothing, commodes and urine bottles as appropriate. **Not being able to get out of the chair** is a common cause of incontinence.

Incontinence of faeces

Loss of either solid or runny unformed stools, or soiling of clothing, is referred to as faecal incontinence. Although this is not nearly as common as urinary incontinence it can be far more distressing because of the resulting mess and smell.

The most common cause is severe constipation, which can happen in children as well as adults, when a hard mass of stool forms in the the lower part of the bowel (see diagram below). Liquid stool trickles past the blockage as a continual faecal loss, causing soiling of clothes and bedding. This is called **constipation with overflow**. It has a very distinctive smell and should not be confused with soiling because the child or adult has not been able to clean themselves, or diarrhoea due to tummy upset or allergy.

There are many causes: embarrassment at using a strange lavatory, poor diet including insufficient fluids, lack of exercise, certain medicines, difficulty in passing hard lumps or a solid mass, or an interruption of the nerve messages to the brain such as occurs in spinal injury or spina bifida.

The simple management is to avoid the situation by ensuring that the toilets are acceptable, the diet is adequate, and a routine is established. The best time for a bowel movement is very individual but after a meal or hot drink, when the gut

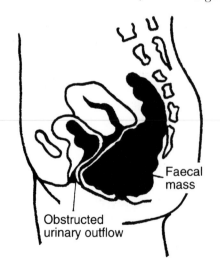

Side view of female showing how constipation can affect the bladder outflow and cause incontinence of urine.

has been stimulated, is often good.

Bulking and softening agents, suppositories, and in extreme cases an enema to clear out the bowel, may be necessary. It will be a medical or nursing decision, but you have an important part in contributing to this.

Young children can find constipation very frightening and upsetting as well as painful if the stool is particularly hard or large. They may try to prevent themselves having a bowel movement or may well use this as a means of attracting attention. Whatever the reason it is important that the situation is treated in the early stages.

In the ageing bowel the sphincter muscles may become lax and less efficient, or there may be a lifetime of straining to open the bowels or a persistent use of laxatives which contribute to the loss of control. In most cases the symptoms can be treated. New techniques in surgery can sometimes improve the function of the muscles controlling the back passage, which may have been damaged at birth or as the result of an injury.

Bowels are a very private affair and should be dealt with discreetly. If protective garments are necessary they should be snug fitting to avoid seepage. Special attention must be given to skin care and personal hygiene; in severe cases it may be necessary to provide a deodorising agent to maintain the client's dignity.

Toileting programme

Toileting is the term applied to the intervals when clients should visit or be taken to the lavatory to maintain bladder and bowel control. The programme will depend on several factors including the bladder function, mental ability and mobility of the client. Clients must be assessed as individuals so that the most appropriate programme can be introduced.

Toileting cannot be imposed on an unwilling or uncooperative client, even if they are intellectually competent. It is therefore important that client and staff alike are convinced that success is achievable.

The assessment will include keeping accurate charts of the times urine is passed in each 24 hours, and the amount if possible. This record should be kept for five to seven days so that a pattern may emerge on which to base the programme. This requires the motivation and cooperation of all staff as well as the client. Whenever possible encourage the client to fill in the record themselves. Many commercial companies provide simple easy-to-record charts and children have great fun creating their own imaginative charts.

It is important that both clients and staff understand what is expected of them, and then stick to the programme.

Set interval toileting is reminding or taking the client to the toilet. It does not teach independence but is useful for people who forget, have no bladder sensation or have no regular pattern of passing urine.

Individualised toileting is working out when the client is most likely to pass urine, by following the chart you made, and then reminding, or taking them to the lavatory 15 minutes before wetting may occur, and adjusting the time interval as necessary.

Bladder retraining is a programme to extend the intervals between going to pass urine. The aim is to hold on for two- to three-hourly intervals. It is useful for people who have lost their confidence and go just in case, but it does need much understanding and support for client and helper.

Personal protection

Sometimes it may be necessary to provide protective garments or appliances for clients who are not able to be completely dry or who are awaiting treatment.

There are thousands of aids available which can make selection difficult. The final choice of product must be made by the client whenever possible, but the type of product will depend on the nature of the incontinence – urinary, faecal or both; the quantity of loss – leak, gush or soiling; the personal details of the client including sex, dexterity, mobility and mental ability.

If reusables are to be tried the laundry facilities need to be flexible to allow for the manufacturer's washing instructions. The availability of the product once the client goes home is most important.

Washing sheets and clothing is difficult and needs to be very carefully considered and incorporated into the care plan. Family carers who are not in the best of health themselves will need help.

You should aim to become as familiar as possible with the products used, their application and management, so that you can advise and support your client and relatives as well as provide a high quality of care. Too often aids are inappropriate, or are used incorrectly because of ignorance or lack of instruction. This can be costly to the client's dignity as well as your time and the resources of the unit.

The continence adviser can advise on selection, although this is often restricted by cost and local purchasing policies. Some products are expensive for regular use if bought independently.

Pads and pants
Absorbent garments and pads are the most commonly used, and reusable products are becoming popular for people who have a long term urinary loss. They

are not recommended for a faecal loss because of staining and washing difficulties. An absorbent aid is designed to keep a client comfortable and free from leakage for 3-4 hours.

For men and women who have a light loss, machine washable pants with an absorbent gusset can give a feeling of confidence. Where the loss is more severe, there is a range of disposable or reusable liners which can be worn inside the person's own pants.

Body worn liners should be cupped to form a gully, with the absorbent surface facing upwards and kept in position with close fitting pants.

Pants and all-in-one garments should be selected by hip fitting. Check the manufacturer's instructions if you are uncertain. Do make sure the user and carer at home understand how to use the product, dispose of soiled pads and how supplies are obtained. Many authorities have a computerised system which automatically allocates a regular supply and reassessment.

Sheaths: Men may prefer to wear an appliance such as a disposable sheath, which should remain in position for 24 hours. There are other appliances which can be worn for longer periods. The initial sizing and fitting should be under the supervision of a nurse or appliance practitioner. These products are available on prescription from the GP. Little boys and older men who have a retracted penis may have difficulty keeping disposable sheaths on, and should be offered an alternative.

Sheets: There are also highly absorbent washable bed sheets which can help to improve sleep patterns because they keep the person warm and dry. It is important to follow the manufacturer's instructions

to obtain the maximum benefit, and check the client's laundry facilities as an automatic washing machine with a range of wash temperatures is essential.

Catheter care

Sometimes a hollow tube called a catheter is placed in the bladder in order to drain the urine away. A catheter may be used once and then removed (intermittent catheterisation) or left in position to drain continuously and changed at intervals (indwelling catheter).

Intermittent catheterisation is passing a fine, usually plastic, catheter through the urethra into the bladder to completely drain it of urine at regular intervals. Children can be taught at a very early age and likewise for adults old age is no barrier, but sight, dexterity and willingness are important.

This method of bladder control has revolutionised the lives of people of all ages who had previously suffered repeated urinary infections and had their lifestyle severely restricted. It is suitable for clients whose bladder is unable to empty completely for some reason, such as children with spina bifida and adults with multiple sclerosis. Whenever possible the client is encouraged to catheterise themselves, so that they are more independent.

The indwelling catheter is passed in to the bladder, usually through the urethra, but sometimes directly into the bladder via the abdomen. It is made of a latex or silicone material, depending on the length of time it is to remain in the bladder, and is attached to a drainage bag, which collects the urine. It is important always to ensure that the connecting tubing is not kinked or compressed so that the urine can flow freely, and that the bag is below the level of the bladder, as urine cannot flow uphill.

The bag can be supported by leg straps or a garment such as a pouch sewn on to the leg of underpants or trousers. The method of support is important as it not only assists in the drainage but also in the dignity of the client. No one likes to see bags of urine and many clients do not want their family and friends to know this intimate aspect of their care.

Clients and relatives can find the prospect of a catheter daunting and you may find yourself having to allay their fears, by explaining clearly so they understand the reasons and the care of the system. Most of the catheter manufacturers provide excellent client guides.

Any indication of infection, such as the client feeling ill or having a raised temperature, should be reported to nursing staff immediately. Clients should also have a contact name and telephone number for emergencies such as a blocked catheter.

Hygiene guidelines

• Always wash hands before as well as after emptying the drainage bag.

• Attach the night bag to the leg bag rather than changing one to the other.

• Never allow the tap of the drainage bag to touch the floor.

• Pay special attention to personal hygiene and washing between the legs.

• Ensure that the catheter and drainage tube are draining freely, and there is no blockage.

• The bag should slope towards the tap to allow complete emptying.

• Support and maintain the shape of the bag using a garment or straps. Remember legs can become swollen by evening so check straps have not become too tight, or hang the bag on a stand on the wheelchair or bed.

Sex

Incontinence can have a devastating effect on relationships. As many people are sexually active in their 70s and 80s it is important to let them know that they can continue to have intercourse.

Reassure them that a catheter can remain in place, but the drainage bag should be emptied first and secured to the leg or tummy. A sheath or similar appliance should be removed first. Assure them that urine is not infectious, and advise them that an absorbent sheet placed under the couple will act as a precaution and give greater confidence.

Stoma care

A "stoma" is the term used when a part of the bowel or tubes leading from the bladder are surgically brought out onto the abdominal wall because of disease. Colostomies and ileostomies carry faeces to a collecting bag attached to the skin on the abdomen. Urostomies carry urine. The site of the stoma and collecting appliance must be looked after carefully in the first few weeks after surgery.

People will usually be taught in hospital to care for their stoma and to apply and change collecting appliances. They may also require further help to overcome the psychological stress of having a stoma or need assistance with physically applying and changing the appliances.

Fears and anxieties

People with stomas naturally have a number of fears and anxieties and it is important to discuss these. Often people need as much help to overcome fears and anxieties as physical help with fitting a stoma appliance. Many hospitals, community health services and manufacturers of stoma appliances will also have specialist nurses who can be called upon for expert advice and guidance in stoma care, such as how to get stoma bags on prescription. You can help by listening to people's worries and repeating any advice and information given by these experts.

Many people fear that they will not be able carry on working or playing sports. In addition people have an altered image of themselves: they fear that their stoma will be noticeable to everyone or that they will no longer be sexually attractive to other people. People can be supported through this period by assuring them that they can continue with their normal lifestyle, including sexual activity, and helping them to manage in the same way that we all manage our own personal toilet needs.

A common fear people have is that they will smell. Stoma appliances are usually odour free if fitted correctly, and charcoal filters and deodorisers are available with certain appliances.

Food and drink

All individuals with a stoma will normally be encouraged to eat a wide variety of foods. Some foods may however cause diarrhoea and excess flatulence. One way of overcoming this may be to take smaller amounts of a particular food, rather than give it up altogether. In addition certain foods are digested more slowly and it will help to ensure that they are chewed well in order to reduce the work of the stomach and intestines.

There are no dietary restrictions for people with a urostomy, but some clients may not drink their normal amounts of fluids in order to reduce the number of times that their appliance bag is changed. An adequate and normal amount of fluids should always be encouraged.

Choosing an appliance

A qualified member of staff should always be responsible for assessing people and fitting stoma appliances in the first few days of care. Appliances are labelled according to the size of the opening that fits around the stoma and a measuring guide for correct choice is usually made available with the appliance. To keep the skin undamaged the stoma must be protected from the adhesive and bag. The appliance should therefore fit snugly around to within 0.5 cm of the stoma edge.

Appliances now widely used are designed to be leak and odour proof, unobtrusive, noiseless and disposable.As a general rule they fall into two categories:
• One piece appliances comprise a bag with an adhesive attached to it. The bag and the adhesive are removed when the appliance is changed.
• Two piece appliances consist of a *flange* that adheres to the skin and a bag that clips onto the flange. This method means that the adhesive can be changed less frequently and helps to protect the skin.

Stoma accessories
Mild soap and water is all that is required for cleaning the skin. Creams and skin barriers should only be used if these are designed specifically for people with stomas. Lotions, sprays and gels, protective wafers and rings are also available to protect the skin around the stoma. Again these should only be used where the advice of a qualified member of staff or a stoma therapist has been sought.

Points to remember

1. You are central in reassuring clients that their problems are recognised and will be given sympathetic help.

2. Your knowledge will give you the confidence to encourage clients to talk about their problems. Ask senior staff if you feel unsure about a query or problem.

3. Bladder and bowel control (continence) is a skill we learn in early life and normally retain till the end.

4. Losing this control – incontinence – is nevertheless a very common problem.

5. The symptoms are embarrassing for clients and care workers alike. It is not an easy subject to talk about: recognising your own feelings is important.

6. Incontinence is a symptom which has many causes.

7. Incontinence can often be cured, and always improved.

8. Success depends on the accurate recording and reporting of your observations to the team.

9. Treatment is a team effort involving the client, their family and all care staff.

10. Attention to the fears and worries of people with incontinence or a stoma is at least as important as their physical care.

Resources

Caring for Continence by Mandy Fader and Christine Norton. Practical guide for care assistants. *Better Care Guides* series, Hawker Publications (1994) London.

Incontinence and Inappropriate Urinating by Graham Stokes. Winslow Press (1994) Bicester.

Incontinence Helpline Disability North at the Dene Centre, Castle Farm Road, Newcastle-upon-Tyne NE3 1PH. Helpline: 091 213 0050, weekdays 9am - 6pm.

Association for Continence Advice, 2 Doughty Street London WC1 2PH. Tel: 071 404 6821. Multi-disciplinary organisation for professionals. **InconTact,** at the same address, is a consumer-led organisation offering information and support for people with bladder and bowel problems.

ERIC: Enuresis Resource Information Centre, 65 St Michael's Hill, Bristol BS2 8DZ. Tel: 0272 264920. Provides information on day and night-time wetting to children, their parents and professionals.

British Colostomy Association, 38-39 Eccleston Square, London SW1V 1PB. Tel: 071 828 5175.

British Digestive Foundation, 3 St Andrew's Place, Regents Park, London NW1 4LB. Tel: 071 487 5332.

Ileostomy Association of Great Britain and Ireland, PO Box 23, Mansfield, Nottinghamshire NG18 4TT. Tel: 0623 28099.

Urostomy Association, Buckland, Beaumont Park, Danbury, Essex CM3 4DE. Tel: 0245 224294.

NVQ Level 2 & 3 Core Units
O Promote equality for all individuals.
U4 Contribute to the health, safety and security of individuals and their environment.
U5 Obtain, transmit and store information relating to the delivery of a care service.
Level 2 Core Unit
W2 Contribute to the ongoing support of clients and others significant to them.
Level 3 Core Unit
Y2 Enable clients to make use of available services and information.
Level 2 Direct Care
Z6 Enable clients to maintain and improve their mobility.
Z9 Enable clients to maintain their personal hygiene and appearance.
Z11 Enable clients to access and use toilet facilities.
Z19 Enable clients to achieve physical comfort.

CHAPTER 19

Drugs, medicines and homely remedies

Sally Shulman

- *Medicines help many people stay independent* • *The supply of medicines*
- *What else should you know?* • *Compliance aids and monitored dose systems*
- *Contra-indications and side effects* • *Over the counter and homely medicines*

Medicines are an essential part of the lives of many people, and giving medicines, or helping people to take them, is important in enabling individuals to remain independent in their own homes.

Medicines (or drugs) are used for a number of reasons. They can treat symptoms, cure disease, replace a missing body substance, or prevent symptoms or illness. Although a qualified member of staff should ultimately be responsible for assessing care needs including the administration of medicines, you as a care assistant will be involved in the day-to-day administering of medicines, applying creams and lotions or instilling ear or eye drops. You may simply be required to supervise clients when they take their medication, or you might have to administer the medicines if the client is unable to do so.

It is important that you feel competent to carry out delegated tasks involving medication, and it is a good idea to obtain some practical training beforehand. The training should cover the storing and correct administration of medicines, and will give you the knowledge and confidence to seek professional advice if you think some-thing is wrong. Initially, you should be supervised and assessed by a senior member of staff, to make sure that you are following instructions, and administering the medicines correctly.

Medicines policy

When a care assistant has to administer or look after medicines as part of their job, there should be a local medicines policy. The medicines policy describes the arrangements for the handling of medicines, including their supply, storage and disposal, as well as administration and record keeping procedures.

The policy covers legal and professional requirements of the organisation employing you, and maintains a safe, effective medicines service for the client. It ensures that care is the same even if there is a change of staff, and protects staff who carefully follow the policy from a claim of negligence should something go wrong.

Supply of medicines

Medicines are prescribed by the doctor for the client according to individual needs.

148

If the client is in hospital, those medicines are ordered by the nurse or the pharmacist, as described in the local policy. In the community, the policy will say who should order and collect prescriptions for clients.

As a care assistant, you will need to know:
• how long the client should use each medicine
• when the medicine will run out
• how to send the doctor a written order for the prescription. There may be a repeat prescription card, book, or computer slip.

The responsible person should:
• send or take the order to the surgery about a week before the medicines run out
• two days later, collect the prescription and take it to the client's usual pharmacy (chemist)
• collect the medicines
• check the labels on the medicines.
The details should agree with the labels on the clients' old medicine bottle, and on the medicines records. If they don't, check whether the doctor has altered the medicines. If not, contact the pharmacist for advice at once.
• enter the quantity of medicine received on the medicines record. Contact the pharmacist for advice if the client runs out of medicine before you get a prescription.

Storage of medicines
• Store medicines securely and out of the reach of children. The medicines policy may specify locked storage cupboards.
• Store medicines in a cool dry place. (Not in the fridge unless the label says so). The pharmacist can advise you.
• Store medicines in the container supplied by the pharmacist. This will be correctly labelled, and suitable to keep the medicine in good condition.

Disposal of medicines
Medicines should be disposed of if the client's requirements change, or the treatment is completed. Do not use medicines after the expiry date has passed. For safety and security, most local policies ask you to sign for and witness the disposal of medicines. Dispose of all unwanted medicines as described in the policy, or the local pharmacy can dispose of medicines safely for you. They should never be put in the dustbin. Never hoard medicines. They may lose their strength or decompose. Never give prescribed medicines to someone else.

Medicine records and documentation
Records are kept as a security check, and to ensure that clients receive their medicines correctly and safely. The medicines policy will state which records must be kept, and who is responsible for them. Recording the doses enables anyone to see what medication has been given and when.

Master medicines record
Each client has a personal medicines record, which lists all their medication. It will specify the name of each medicine, the strength in milligrammes, the dose, and the times when each medicine should be taken. All other records, charts, or labels on medicines should correspond with the master medicines record. It is important that this is kept up to date and amended as the needs of the client change. Records for ordering, receipt and disposal of medicines may be on the master record, on another chart, or in a book.

Administration of medicines record
A care assistant who is responsible for administering medicines must record each dose. You must record if the client refuses a medicine or if it is not given.

A typical medicine label

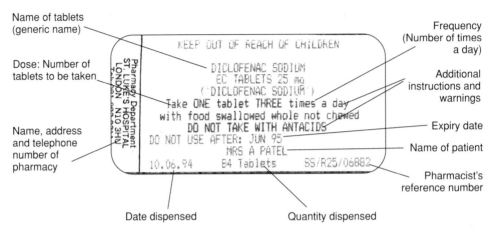

Name of tablets
(generic name)

Dose: Number of
tablets to be taken

Name, address
and telephone
number of
pharmacy

Frequency
(Number of times
a day)

Additional
instructions and
warnings

Expiry date

Name of patient

Pharmacist's
reference number

Date dispensed

Quantity dispensed

Diclofenac is an anti-inflammatory drug. Its brand name is Voltarol. They are both the same drug, different manufacturer.

What else should you know?

• Does it have another name?
Medicines have a trade name, and an official or generic name. Hospitals usually give medicines the official name but GPs may use either. Sometimes a client may have two bottles of the same medicine, with different names, and may take both by mistake. An example is paracetamol (official name). Panadol and Hedex are trade names of paracetamol. Co-proxamol, Lemsip, and Paracodol are trade names of medicines that contain paracetamol as well as other ingredients. Check with the pharmacist if in doubt.

• What is it for? Especially if it is prescribed to be taken "when necessary".

How important is it for the client to take the medicine?

• How long should it be taken for, and when will it run out? Is it a course that should be finished, or does the client need to get a new prescription when it finishes?

Will the doctor need to see the client before giving another prescription?

• Should the client avoid any foods, drinks or other medicines, including those bought from the chemist or health food store?

• Are there any special storage instructions?

• Are there any common side effects to look out for? Will the client's skills be affected?

Always check the label. Ask the pharmacist if you need more information or if you are worried about something.

Administering medicines

• Hygiene
Before you begin, always wash your hands and keep everything as clean as possible. Remember that hygiene is important in safeguarding both you and the client when touching and administering medicines.

• Check the medicine records
Check that the name of the client corre-

sponds with that on the medicine label. **Never risk giving medicine to the wrong person.** If the client is confused, check their identity with someone who knows them. Make sure you have all the medicines listed on the record.

• **Check the label**
If the print is not clear, take the bottle back to the chemist who supplied it.

Check the name of the client, the date or expiry date on the label, the name and strength of the medicine, and the instructions. Check any extra labels, which give advice or warnings about the medicine.

• **Explain the procedure**
Make sure the client knows what to do, or what to expect.

• **Administer the medicine**

• **Record whether the medicine is administered or not.** Give reasons if it is not given, for example if the client refuses. Report this to someone in charge.

Compliance aids

Compliance aids are devices that are used to make it easier for clients to administer medicines themselves. For example the "Opticare" helps clients to squeeze and aim eye drops. The "Haleraid" helps clients to squeeze some types of inhaler.

A daily or weekly supply of medicines can also be put out in advance with a compliance aid. The client, perhaps supervised by a carer, takes the medicine from the compartment for the day of the week, and the time of day. The care assistant can look at the empty compartments, to see if the dose has been taken. If the client is not taking the medicines correctly, the care assistant should seek advice.

It is best if a card is attached to the device, labelled with the contents and doses in the device, for example, the "Daily Pill Minder", the "Medidos", or the "Dosette".

Care assistants should not administer medicines from compliance aids, unless they are filled and labelled by the pharmacist.

Medicines that were dispensed and labelled by the pharmacist should be administered directly from the container to avoid mistakes which may occur when medicines and labels are transferred from one container to another.

Monitored dose systems

These can be useful when a number of professional and family carers administer medicines to a client, and they are popular in residential care homes. The medicines are dispensed and sealed by the pharmacist in weekly or monthly packs.

Administering the medication
The care assistant administers the tablet from the compartment labelled with the correct day of the week and correct administration time. Each tablet or capsule can be clearly identified from the label.

The medicine records can be filled in accurately.

If the medication is altered, ask the pharmacist to repack the medicines.

Examples of monitored dose systems include "Nomad", "Venalink", and the "Manrex" (or Boots) system. All these systems are available from many pharmacies.

The medicines policy should include a section on the correct use of compliance aids or monitored dose systems in the organisation.

Contra-indications

There are a number of illnesses where a certain medication should not be used, and the doctor and pharmacist should look out for these.

For example, it is dangerous to give aspirin or certain common arthritis medicines to patients who have had a stomach ulcer, or give beta-blockers such as atenolol to patients with asthma.

Side effects

Side effects are the unwanted effects of medicines.

Common side effects include:

• Drowsiness from antihistamines (drugs for allergy and hay fever), tranquillisers and antidepressants.
• Constipation from codeine (for coughs) and morphine (for pain).
• Headache with glyceryl trinitrate (for angina chest pains).

These side effects almost always occur with these medicines and the chemist should warn the client or carer to expect them.

• Rashes from certain antibiotics, and many other drugs.
• Stomach pain with aspirin and certain arthritis drugs.
• Diarrhoea with antibiotics.

These dangerous side effects only occur in a few people who take these drugs.

Very rarely, side effects can kill or cause serious harm. Blood disorders, allergic reactions, and stomach bleeding are some possible severe side effects.

Side effects and older people

Older people are more likely to suffer side effects, partly because they take more medicines. They are often more sensitive to drugs, and their bodies do not dispose of them so easily. They may suffer dizziness, confusion, coughing, dry mouth, difficulty in passing urine, too frequent passing of urine, or agitation, among others.

Avoiding side effects

Sometimes a side effect can be avoided or reduced, or it may gradually disappear of its own accord. Alternatively the doctor might alter the dose or time of administration, or change the drug to one that better suits the client. However, sometimes side effects are unavoidable, and the client will have to accept them.

What should you do?

Find out the common side effects of the drugs your client is on, and keep a lookout for changes in the client's normal condition. Make a note of any changes, and tell a qualified member of staff if you feel there is cause for concern. If no one is available the client's regular pharmacist may be able to advise you.

Some drugs can be harmful if they are stopped suddenly, so seek medical advice. Your local policy will state if you should contact the doctor.

Homely medicines

The client can buy "over the counter" medicines from the chemist without a prescription. They may be used to treat mild symptoms such as colds, constipation or headaches. The pharmacist can recommend a remedy that the client can take safely with their other medicines, or will advise if they should see a doctor. The pharmacist can check whether the symptoms are caused by a side effect of another medicine. As a care assistant, **you should never recommend a remedy,** and you should only give medicines if they are prescribed by the doctor.

If someone else gives the client an "over the counter" remedy, check with the client's pharmacist that it is suitable. Record any "over the counter" remedies that the client is taking.

A homely remedies policy is found in some organisations such as care homes. A homely remedies policy will describe:

• A small list of "over the counter medicines", that can be kept.
• The dose of each medicine.

• The symptoms for which each medicine can be given. For example mild pain, indigestion, coughs, and constipation.

• Any extra advice on treating the symptoms.

• The number of days it can be given, before a doctor is called.

Only senior designated staff will be allowed to decide if a homely remedy should be administered to a client. The policy should be agreed with the pharmacist and doctor.

If homely remedies are administered, records should be made.

Points to remember

1. Follow your local Medicines Policy. Keep medicines records up to date, to protect the client and you.

2. Make sure the client's regular medicines don't run out. Use the client's regular chemist (pharmacist).

3. Store medicines safely and securely. Follow any special storage instructions from the pharmacist.

4. Always administer medicines from the original container, labelled by the pharmacist. Do not transfer medicines into another container.

5. Always read the labels on medicine containers. Check the client's name, the medicine's name and strength, and the dose to be given.

6. Check that compliance aids or monitored dose systems are used correctly. Only administer medicines from these if the pharmacist has filled and clearly labelled them.

7. Look out for side effects of medicines, or changes in the client's condition. Report them to a qualified person, and make a record.

8. Make a record if clients in the community wish to use "over the counter" medicines or homely remedies. Always check with the regular pharmacist, who can advise if the remedy is suitable.

9. If you have any concerns about medicines, always check with your manager, a nurse, a pharmacist, or the doctor. Who you check with first, depends on the situation and on your local policy.

Further reading

For information with diagrams, on different kinds of medicines and how to administer them, and on commonly used medicines and their side effects:
Using Medicines: A guide for the professional carer. Alan Humfress, Senior Pharmacist, St Lukes Hospital, Woodside Avenue, London N10 3HU.

NVQ Level 2 & 3 Core Units

O Promote equality for all individuals.

Z1 Contribute to the protection of individuals from abuse.

U4 Contribute to the health, safety and securityand individuals an their environment.

U5 Obtain, transmit and store information relating to the delivery of a care service.

Level 2 Core Unit

W2 Contribute to the ongoing support of clients and others significant to them.

Level 3 Core Unit

Y2 Enable clients to make use of available services and information.

Level 2 Domiciliary Support

U1 Contribute to the maintenance and management of domestic and personal resources.

CHAPTER 20

Inappropriate and aggressive behaviour

Valerie Good

• What is inappropriate? • Three golden rules • Prevention
• When it happens • Coping with violence and aggression • Coping with
inappropriate sexual behaviour

Most care assistants will sooner or later work with a client who behaves in a way that is unacceptable, embarrassing or frightening. This chapter includes advice on how to reduce the likelihood of this kind of behaviour happening, coping with the behaviour if it occurs and what to do after any incident. Some of the advice will apply no matter what the behaviour is; other advice will relate to particular specific situations.

What is inappropriate?

Everybody has a different view of what kind of behaviour can be called "inappropriate" and what kind of behaviour makes them feel distressed or threatened. Your tolerance and your responses will have been shaped by your upbringing and by the experiences that you have faced during your life. As a care assistant you will have to decide what you find acceptable and manageable and what you find offensive and intolerable; it is not something that can be laid down by your managers in a policy or a handbook.

The most common form of unaccept-

able behaviour relates to some sort of aggressive act. The aggression may take the form of verbal abuse, threats or actual attempts to harm you. Unacceptable behaviour also includes inappropriate sexual conduct such as a client making sexual remarks or advances to you or masturbating in front of you.

Sometimes you will be assisting someone you know well and the unacceptable behaviour will come "out of the blue" and will appear to be completely out of character. On other occasions you may be asked to help someone who has a reputation for being "difficult" and you will be half expecting trouble. Regardless of whether the behaviour is expected or not there are some key points to bear in mind.

Three golden rules

1. Know yourself
As a care worker it is important for you to be aware of yourself and have an understanding of how you may react in different situations. Are you naturally trusting, always wanting to believe the best of people? Or are you more cynical, finding it easy to find fault with people. You should

aim to take a balanced view, where difficulties are not expected at every turn but where you are sensitive to the possibility of dangers and difficulties.

You should also think about how you react to stress or aggression. Would you categorise yourself as someone who "stands their ground", as someone "who turns and runs" or as someone who gets "frozen to the spot"?

2. Know the client

Coping with inappropriate behaviour must include looking at what you do before visiting a new client. It is important to know as much as you can about the person you are going to visit. The amount of information available to you will vary but you should always take the opportunity to talk to your manager and read the care plan. You need details about why the person needs help and about any preferences they have about the way they are assisted.

You must try not to pigeonhole new clients into stereotypes: not all people who are mentally ill will be unstable and unpredictable and not all "old ladies of 90" will be grateful and passive.

3. Understand the causes of unacceptable behaviour

Understanding some of the reasons why a client may act in a particular way may help you avoid having to cope with the behaviour and may help you find ways of managing the situation.

The causes fall into three broad groups:

Pain and stress: Most people who are in pain find themselves short tempered and less tolerant than normal. This will apply to many clients who are either coping with chronic pain or who have sudden episodes of ill health. Other clients will live in stressful situations caused by poor housing, poverty, or unhappy and unfulfilling relationships. Anger and resentment can build up and lead to an outburst of aggression, or the episode of unacceptable behaviour may be the client's way of trying to get you to recognise their distress.

The last straw: Sometimes the behaviour you see may have little connection with you or what you have done. The client may have had a series of things happen to them before you visit; they may have had a row with a family member, a "final demand" in the post or a sleepless night. You may be the first person to visit after this and you may say or do something that would normally be unremarkable but the client's reaction is extreme.

Misunderstanding: There will be some clients who misunderstand what is said or done or misinterpret what they see. They may then react in a way that appears irrational or bizarre. This kind of situation may arise when the client has impaired sight or hearing, has a learning disability, is confused or is hallucinating.

Prevention

Minimising the chance of unacceptable behaviour occurring

As a care assistant working in the community you need to always be aware that you are a visitor in someone else's home. You should be always courteous and ask permission before undertaking tasks. The client should always be consulted about how and when things should be done. There are several things you should bear in mind:

It's not what you say it's the way that you say it

We all have "give away" signs that indicate a range of emotions, such as feeling tense, anxious or relaxed. If you pay attention to the client's body language you should be able to tell when they are getting angry or upset. It is equally important that you are aware of the messages your body language and tone of voice give to the client. Can they tell from your manner that you think that they are a nuisance or that you dislike working with them?

You will have read in an earlier chapter about talking and listening skills; these should help you pick up clues about how the client is feeling and help ensure that you can be clearly understood without sounding patronising.

Give people space and time

Most care assistants have busy schedules and there is a great temptation to rush and bustle around a client's home. It is important that you always make time, particularly when you first arrive, to talk to the client about how they are and what they want you to do. Sometimes clients will appear agitated or distressed and it will be more important for you to give them your full attention rather than "getting on" with your normal routine.

It is helpful if you can be sensitive to people's personal space. Two common faults are standing too close, or standing towering over someone who is seated. Both can feel intimidating and lead to a client acting aggressively.

Be aware of trigger points

If you are working with someone who you know may behave in an aggressive or inappropriate way you may be able to work out what kind of things trigger the behaviour. It could be that particular things you say remind the client of someone else, or the client may find your dress or behaviour provocative.

When it happens

If you think that a situation is becoming intolerable or getting out of hand then it is up to you to act, and you must trust your own judgement. There will be some situations when all that is necessary is for you to tell the client clearly that you want them to stop what they are doing. At other times it will be necessary to remove yourself from the situation.

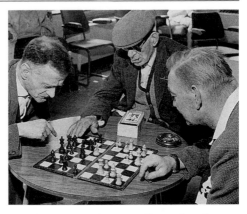

Don't pigeonhole: not all people who are mentally ill will be unstable and unpredictable.

Saying no

In some situations it will be possible to negotiate with the client about the behaviour, by saying something like:

"I don't want you to do that while I am here."

It is important that you act confidently and don't appear to be the victim. It is much better to say "I want you to stop that immediately" rather than "Please don't do that." It is also vital that you do not promise anything that you can't deliver or make any ultimatums that cannot be enforced. For example it would be unwise to say "if you behave yourself I'll get the day centre to let you go on the trip" or "if you do that I'll make sure that you don't get any more help".

Keeping calm

When you are upset or distressed it is easy to respond aggressively, or to speak sharply. You have a responsibility as a care worker to try to stay calm and to resist the temptation to retaliate. You may find it helpful to take several deep breaths and count to ten before you say or do anything.

Never threaten, or invite retaliation from someone.

Getting out

There will be rare occasions where you feel unsafe in a situation and want to leave. This may just mean a five minute break in another room while everyone cools off, at other times it will involve leaving completely. When visiting a new client it is worthwhile noting the layout of their home and ensuring that you can identify the "escape routes".

If you are being held or the client is blocking the escape route you may have to use force. The best advice is to "bash and dash". The targets to aim for, with a kick, are the shin or knee. A hard twist to the cheeks, nose or ears is always painful as well. It is often suggested that women should aim a knee in the groin of any man who is threatening them, but this is not a good tactic, as it puts you off balance, making you vulnerable.

You may think that this is all very extreme, and you may never need to take such action. However it may be worth spending half an hour practising some of these skills with colleagues. You could also ask your manager if there is any appropriate training or policy on violence and aggression available.

Afterwards

If the incident has upset you, consider whether it is a good idea to go on to your next visit or whether you need time to recover. You have a responsibility to report the incident to your manager straight away. You need to describe the circumstances leading up to the situation, what happened and how you responded. This should be done clearly and without exaggerating. It is much more helpful to say "Mr Jones threatened me with his clenched fist when I asked him to move to another chair" rather than "I was only helping him and he was violent towards me". You should also make sure that you have an opportunity to discuss your feelings with someone appropriate.

Reporting an incident is not the same as admitting defeat and it may help protect other workers by forewarning them about the situation.

If you have been in this situation already, you will be able to recall how you felt. You may have felt a failure, thinking that as a caring person you ought to be able to cope. You may not have told your manager about what happened, either seeing it as a sign of weakness, or because you thought it might lead to the client being labelled as dangerous or aggressive. All of these reactions are understandable, but do not help you, the client or other colleagues.

You need to make the time to reflect on what happened, and you may want to discuss with your manager about whether you go back to the client. If you do wish to go back, you will need to talk about what needs to be changed to avoid the same situation reoccurring.

Coping with violence and aggression

The mildest forms of aggression are swearing and verbal abuse. This may include racial and sexual harassment. It is hard to find a commonly accepted definition of abuse but you should include anything that makes *you* feel as if you have been abused.

Care assistants need to be able to tell the difference between aggression and assertiveness in clients. The client has the right to express their opinions and views but not to be abusive towards you. Sometimes the gender of the aggressor or abuser will make a difference; if you are a woman you may feel more frightened of an aggressive man but more surprised by an abusive outburst from a woman.

Responding to aggression with aggression will only lead to more violence. You should try to lower the emotional temperature instead, and stay calm, speak slowly and clearly and not argue. It is not usually a good idea to try to touch the person or to try to keep continual eye contact with them. Be particularly aware of your body language – are your hands on your hips and are you pointing your finger accusingly?

If you are working with a client who is occasionally aggressive you should bear in mind that there are some rooms in a house that hold more dangers than others – it may make sense to avoid having disagreements in the kitchen! It is also a wise precaution to make sure that someone knows where you are and your expected times of arrival and departure.

Coping with inappropriate sexual behaviour

Many care assistants will find inappropriate sexual behaviour harder to cope with than threats or abuse. Part of the problem is that some people find it difficult to talk about incidents that have a sexual connotation. If this applies to you it is worth considering ways of overcoming you embarrassment.

Some inappropriate behaviour may be caused by the client misinterpreting the way you dress, and the way you speak to them or touch them. You may think that calling them "dear" or giving them a hug is harmless or that flirting with them will "cheer them up", but it may lead some people to fantasise that there is more to the relationship.

Particular care needs to be taken if you are providing personal care such as assisting people to bathe or use the toilet. You should take care to treat the person with dignity, give them as much privacy as possible and never tease or joke about them or the situation unless you are absolutely certain about their response. If you are working with someone with a learning disability you may need to check with your manager about the kind of sex education they have

had and the extent of their understanding.

Points to remember

1. Be prepared: the more you know about the client's background, the better you'll be able to cope.
2. Remember at all times that you are a visitor in someone's home.
3. Be aware of the client's and your own body language.
4. Give people time and space.
5. Never retaliate, either by arguing or threatening.
6. Trust your own judgement; leave if you feel unsafe.
7. Report all incidents to your manager and take the opportunity to discuss your feelings about what has happened.
8. Do not tease or flirt with clients.
9. Be aware of dangers but don't look for trouble.

Further reading
Royal College of Nursing (1994) *Violence and Community Nursing Staff. Advice for Nurses.*

NVQ Level 2 & 3 Core Units
O Promote equality for all individuals.
Z1 Contribute to the protection of individuals from abuse.
U4 Contribute to the health, safety and security of individuals and their environment.
U5 Obtain, transmit and store information relating to the delivery of a care service.

Level 2 Core Unit
W2 Contribute to the ongoing support of clients and others significant to them.

Level 3 Core Units
Z3 Contribute to the management of aggressive and abusive behaviour.
Z4 Promote communication with clients where there are communication difficulties.
Z8 Support clients when they are distressed.
Y2 Enable clients to make use of available services and information.

Level 2 Domiciliary Support
W8 Enable clients to maintain contacts in potentially isolating situations.

CHAPTER 21

Abuse and inadequate care

Stuart Darby

• Who is abused? • Different types of abuse and contributing factors • Identifying abuse • Your role • Reporting incidents of abuse • Participating in investigations • Helping and supporting carers • Preventing abuse

Most people are able to live independently at home, or with the help and assistance of relatives, friends, neighbours or health and social service workers. However, for a proportion of people receiving care from others this may cause conflict. It may lead to them being exploited and may mean that abuse and inadequate care takes place.

People who are abused or who receive inadequate care are most likely to be those who are dependent, and cannot "escape" from their situation because they have physical, mental or emotional difficulties. They may be reliant upon another person, a carer, to help them with a number of their physical acts of daily living, such as washing, shopping and cooking or they may be unable to cope with essential tasks such as understanding and managing their finances. For some people escaping from the situation may not be an easy option. They may prefer to live with the abuse rather than move to a residential or nursing home.

Conversely, some carers can also be abused by the very people for whom they provide care. They may feel duty bound to look after a dependent parent or partner. When the task of caring takes place 24 hours a day, seven days a week, 52 weeks of the year, this can create unbearable demands and become a major burden. The dependent person can often knowingly or unwittingly make this situation worse by refusing to help with their own care or by being physically and verbally obstructive, demanding and demonstrative.

What is abuse?

It is very difficult to define abuse and inadequate care. Some people refuse to acknowledge that it can exist at all, and what seems to be abuse and inadequate care to one person, may not be to another. For example, giving medicine to help a person to sleep may be normal if it is the correct medicine, correct dose and given at the right time. Giving too much of the same medicine at the wrong time however, presents a different picture.

In order to simplify a number of differ-

159

ent definitions, abuse and inadequate care will be described here as:

"Physical, verbal, sexual or racial harm or neglect of a person or their property. This harm may be wilful, deliberate and a direct act, or it may be the inability of a carer to provide adequate care that meets all the needs of a dependent person. Abuse and inadequate care can be a single incident or part of a repeated pattern."

Different types of abuse.
Situations of abuse and inadequate care reported to health and social services often have a number of different features. Age Concern (Action on Elder Abuse) has identified seven main categories:
• physical abuse, such as hitting, slapping, pushing and restraining
• emotional and psychological abuse, including blackmail, blaming or swearing
• deprivation of food, heat, clothing and comfort
• forcible isolation
• sexual abuse
• misusing medicines
• misusing money, property or power over another.

Contributing factors

Any person, man or woman, may be abused, but those who are physically, mentally or emotionally dependent on others are the most vulnerable.

Factors in the dependent person
Factors making abuse more likely include: when the person has a physical illness that restricts mobility or causes incontinence; when they have undergone a major personality change or display behavioural problems such as in dementia, confusion or depression; when the person themselves or the person providing care for them has difficulties talking and communicating with each other because of sight, hearing or speech difficulties.

Low income, poor and inadequate housing and strained long-term family relationships coupled with violent behaviour are also common factors. In addition, when the person will only accept care from one person this adds to the burden and strain.

Factors in carers
Factors making carers more likely to abuse include; when carers have suffered an enforced, unplanned change in their personal lives and careers; where they feel exploited and let down by health and social services; where they find it difficult to get others to understand their stress; when they themselves are physically or mentally ill, exhausted or isolated; when they have financial difficulties, other dependents and responsibilities; where they lack privacy and personal space and are abused by the older dependent person themselves. A dependency upon alcohol and drugs has also been noted.

Other risk factors include a historically poor relationship between carer and the dependent person, particularly where there has been a reversal in the role between parent and child.

Identifying abuse
Although there have been very few research studies in the United Kingdom, a number of common physical indicators of abuse have been identified. It is very important not to use these indicators in isolation as a simple checklist. They should be considered with the social and emotional factors of the dependent person, the carer and their living situation. They should also not be confused with

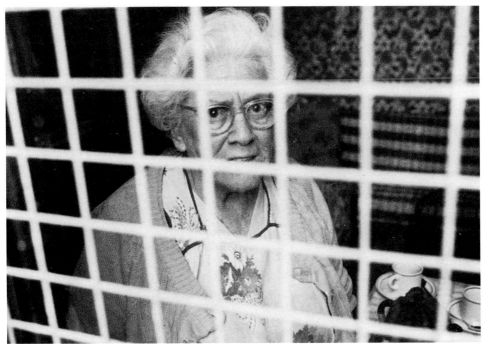

It is very important not to jump to conclusions about possible abuse – discuss your feelings with a qualified member of staff.

genuine accidents or physiological changes of the body associated with getting older.

The following lists have been taken from a number of research studies and reports:

Indicators of physical abuse

• A history of unexplained falls, minor injuries and fractures.

• Pepperpot (knuckle marks) injuries on the chest, and finger marks.

• Unexplained bruises in well protected areas.

• Burns in unusual places.

• Unexplained cuts and lacerations.

• Excessive repeat prescriptions indicating overuse of medicines.

• Underuse of medicines prescribed to treat illness and conditions.

• Excessive consumption of alcohol by carer or older person.

• Bruising and/or bleeding in the genital area and/or venereal disease.

Indicators of inadequate care

• Dehydration.

• Malnutrition.

• Inappropriate clothing (night clothes during the day).

• Poor hygiene, unkempt or unwashed.

• Untreated medical problems.

• Hypothermia.

• Avoidable pressure sores.

• Withdrawn or agitated and anxious.

• They may be isolated in one room of the house.

Social and emotional indicators of abuse in carers.

• Anger, frustration or despair at the situation they are in.

• Resentment of the older dependent person.

- Sense of loss for personal career plans or ambitions.
- Feelings of isolation and loneliness.
- Untreated physical or mental health needs.
- Loss of self value and worth.
- Professional and other visitors may have difficulty getting access to the person.
- The carer always wishes to be present at interviews.
- Poor living accommodation and low income.

Your role

Understanding who is at risk

The most important factor is your knowledge of abuse and inadequate care, who is at risk and how it can occur. It is very important not to jump to conclusions when you encounter a situation that you may not feel comfortable about. Discussing this with a qualified member of staff will help you to concentrate your thoughts and feelings and relate these to your knowledge of what causes abuse and what signs may be present.

Reporting to qualified member of staff

1. It is essential that you always report and discuss your suspicions and concerns about the clients and carers for whom you provide care, to a qualified member of staff as soon as possible. When you have had the opportunity to discuss this, and you both feel confident that an abusing situation may be taking place, you will need to write this down. If you feel that a person is being abused by a colleague, or other paid or voluntary worker, this will need to be investigated by their manager.
2. You should write clearly and accurately the name, age, address, telephone number, gender and first language spoken of the person. It is also useful to note the name of the general practitioner and any other paid worker that you know regularly visits or provides care.
3. If the person has named someone to contact in an emergency, who is not the same person as the abuser you should also note down their name, address, telephone number and relationship.
4. You need to note the alleged abuser's name, relationship, address and telephone number, if you know who this is.
5. Finally, you need to write down a description of the alleged abuse or inadequate care, including the date. This should include any signs that you have observed. In addition you may wish to list the factors that are present that are contributing to the situation. Do not speculate about the abuse. Only write down the facts of what you have seen or heard. You may wish to add descriptions or suspicions of earlier incidents if these were evident. You should give dates of these and any prior action that may have been taken and by whom.

Participating in investigations

It is important that a qualified member of staff or your manager takes responsibility for the investigation from now on. They may feel that the situation is serious enough to report the matter directly to social services and for a social worker to be involved in further investigation. Alternatively they may wish to visit the older person and their carer at home with you, to discuss concerns about their care.

It is important that you are clear about the reason for the visit and that you tell the carer of the concerns and that you wish to help.

At this stage you may be able to help the situation. You may need to offer more support to the person. You may want to refer to other agencies to increase the level and frequency of services or you may wish to consider help for the carer by assisting them to have breaks from caring, for example by arranging day centre care or respite care.

If there are any obvious conditions that require immediate action such as treating injuries, or dealing with personal hygiene or physical needs you should get permission from the person and their carer to carry these out, to ask for the general practitioner to visit or for the person to be referred to hospital.

If the qualified member of staff is not satisfied that the situation can be helped or that it will become worse in the near future they may refer the matter to a social worker. The person and their carer should always be told that this referral is being made.

Continuing to provide care and support

It is important that you continue to provide care and support to the person and their carer. There should be no reason to withdraw care from the home unless you are in physical danger yourself. This can be a very difficult situation, but essentially, while not condoning any abuse or inadequate care, you should be prepared to continue to provide the same or an increased level of support where appropriate and while further investigations are being undertaken.

Contributing to further investigations

Currently, there are no specific laws in the United Kingdom to deal with these types of situations although some health and social services do have local policies. Social workers are the most appropriate care service to investigate alleged abuse. They are also often able to take action to help. In order to do this they may call case conferences and involve other health and social care workers such as general practitioners. On occasions, perhaps where theft or fraudulent use of money is evident, they may need to involve the police. It is important therefore that you keep clear and accurate records of any future visits, and that you keep a copy of your original written report. You may be asked to attend a case conference, which may also include the person, the carer and the alleged abuser if this is not the carer.

Help and support for carers

Carers experience a considerable amount of stress and conflict when they are providing assistance to a dependent older person. They are unable to "switch off" at the end of a day's work, and may be unable to pursue social and leisure activities to take their mind off their caring role. In addition, they may be physically exhausted. Research shows that carers are mostly older women who, because of the demands placed upon them, are unable to seek help with their own physical and emotional health needs. A large part of your continued role may be to listen to and support carers. You may be the only person that they are able to talk to, and as a result they may share many personal thoughts and past experiences with you. It is important that anything that you see or hear remains confidential.

Community Care Assessment

Recent Government legislation recognises the right of everyone to remain in their own homes. It also recognises carers' needs for adequate help to enable them to continue to meet the demands of caring for someone at home.

Under this legislation each person has the right to request a Community Living Assessment. Although the way in which this will take place will differ across the country, the principle is that it provides the opportunity for people to be assessed and to identify their needs to enable them to remain at home. As a care assistant you have an important role to play in directing people to information about appropriate services and agencies who may be able to provide help. This will enable the person and their carer to contribute to any assessment and to ask for the services that will most benefit them. Many of these services will be part of existing and health and social service provision. Some services may also be provided by the independent and voluntary sector, for example Age Concern, Carers National Association or the Alzheimer's Disease Society.

Respite

Carers need to be aware of how to "take a break". This may simply be for a few hours a week, a few days each week or for longer periods of time. "Respite", as this is known, comes in many forms. It may be attendance at a luncheon club, day centre or day hospital. It could also mean admission to a residential or nursing home. These sorts of decisions mostly rest with the person and their carer; your role is to offer information on what is available locally.

Carers groups

Carers groups are often run locally, either by health and social services or by other caring agencies. These meetings provide carers with the opportunity to take a break from the home, to meet others socially as well as the opportunity for carers to discuss their problems. This type of support can be very helpful, particularly where people share information, and their frustrations and how they overcame them.

Counselling

Some carers may feel that they need individual counselling. Many carers have reversed roles, caring for a parent who once cared for them. Others may have given up successful careers to take on caring duties and feel angry and resentful at this change in role. Counselling will enable them to discuss their anxieties and fears in a controlled way, rather than taking it out on the person for whom they are providing care.

Meeting long term needs

Providing care for another person can often go on for many years. Long-term planning needs to take place, perhaps for regular, planned respite, making changes to the home to enable the person to be more independent or make caring easier, providing advice and information on how to claim financial benefits, and providing the opportunity for both the dependent person and carer to seek and receive medical treatment when necessary.

Prevention

Your knowledge of the causes and stresses that can lead to abuse and inadequate care in old age are important factors in preventing it. You may be involved in screening people over the age of seventy-five years as part of a general practitioner's team. This provides you with a good opportunity to identify any stressful situations that people or carers may be having, and to take steps to alleviate them.

Having a knowledge of the "high risk" factors helps to support people and their carers by ensuring appropriate assessment, provision of services and aids and adaptations to the home, and through encouraging independence to help alleviate the physical strain of caring.

By encouraging carers to seek medical help when they need it, and to take the opportunity for regular breaks, you will help to prevent stressful situations leading to abusive situations.

Finally, if you are involved in a situation where abuse and inadequate care is taking place, never reject the person or the carer. Your involvement and support may be the one thing that is keeping a carer going.

Points to remember

1. People who are abused or who receive inadequate care are most likely to be those who are dependent, and cannot "escape" from their situation because they have physical, mental or emotional difficulties.

2. Carers can also be abused by the very people for whom they provide care. The dependent person can often increase the strain by refusing to help with their own care or by being physically and verbally obstructive, demanding and demonstrative.

3. It is important to consider the physical, social and emotional evidence of the dependent person and the alleged abuser, before jumping to conclusions about abuse and inadequate care.

4. Always report and discuss your suspicions and concerns about the clients and carers for whom you provide care, to a qualified member of staff as soon as possible.

5. Making confidential, accurate, legible and complete records is essential.

6. A large part of your role may be to listen to and support carers who may share many personal thoughts and past experiences with you.

7. Continuing to provide sensitive and non-judgemental care where abuse has been disclosed is an important part of supporting clients and carers.

Resources
Bennett G, Kingston P (1993) *Elder abuse: Concepts, theories and interventions.* Chapman Hall, London.
Guidelines on abuse and inadequate care in old age. Royal College of Nursing, London.

Action on Elder Abuse
Age Concern England
Astral House
1268 London Road
London
SW16 4ER
Tel. 081 679 8000

Royal College of Nursing
20, Cavendish Square
London
W1M 0AB
071 409 3333

NVQ Level 2 & 3 Core Units
O Promote equality for all individuals.
Z1 Contribute to the protection of individuals from abuse.
U4 Contribute to the health, safety and security of individuals and their environment.
U5 Obtain, transmit and store information relating to the delivery of a care service.
Level 2 Core Unit
W2 Contribute to the ongoing support of clients and others significant to them.
Level 3 Core Unit
Z3 Contribute to the management of aggressive and abusive behaviour.
Z4 Promote communication with clients where there are communication difficulties.
Z8 Support clients whenthey are distressed.
Y2 Enable clients to make use of available services and information.
Level 2 Domiciliary support
U1 Contribute to the maintenance and management of domestic and personal resources.

CHAPTER 22

Loss, dying and palliative care

Vicky Robinson

• Reactions to loss • Caring for the dying person and their carers at home
• Nursing care • Symptom control • Pain control • Psychological and
emotional care

Palliative care is concerned with providing care to people who are ill and where there is no longer a cure. It aims to enable people to get on with living their lives in comfort, peace and without pain, while they have an illness which will ultimately end their life. Palliative care aims to relieve the suffering of people and their carers who are dying of cancer, HIV disease (AIDS) and other life threatening illnesses.

Reactions to loss

We all face loss of some kind in our lives. This may be through the death of a loved one, loss of a job, a limb, or through other separation such as divorce.

When someone is dying, both they and those close to them are facing very significant loss. As a care assistant working in the community you will be responsible for providing care for people when they are at their most vulnerable.

Although you are accountable to a qualified member of staff, you may sometimes find yourself alone in a situation that you feel ill-equipped to deal with. When looking after dying and bereaved people, it is most important to be honest with ourselves when we find things upsetting. Specialist "palliative" care or "support" teams are available to offer support to community workers to help with practical advice for clients, their carers and staff involved in providing care to those clients who are dying. It is vital to ensure that you get adequate and appropriate support if you find yourself in a situation that is difficult to cope with.

To illustrate how loss can affect people, you may find it helpful to start with the following exercise:

• Think of an object that is very important to you. This object may be a treasured piece of jewellery or a family photograph, or something ordinary like your bed.
• Now imagine that you have just lost it.
• What feelings are you experiencing?
• What are you doing about it?
• Write down your feelings.
• What are you thinking, feeling and doing one day later?
• What are you thinking, feeling and doing a week later when the object is still missing?
• A month has now passed. It is still

missing. What are you thinking, feeling and doing?

• It is six months later. The object has still not been found. What are you thinking, feeling and doing?

• A year later, the object is still missing. What are you thinking, feeling and doing?

Feedback

Your responses to the situations above will be different from those of other people. At the beginning you may feel angry, sad or frightened. You may think continuously about the object, trying to figure out where it could be. Perhaps you spend a lot of time searching for it. As time goes on these reactions usually change. Less and less time is spent thinking about the object and searching for it. Most people begin to accept that the object is gone.

Although uncertainty is part of all of our lives, we are not often conscious of it on a daily basis. The feelings you may have just experienced are an example of how both clients and their families feel at some time during the process of bereavement. We can see that loss applies to many things. For example, the loss of a limb, an organ or a newborn child may give rise to similar emotions.

Peace to explore

Most people, if they are given the choice, prefer to die at home. Those of us working in the community have to make sure that the home is made suitable, providing the right medicines, equipment and essential care without making it into a mini hospital ward.

Clients who are dying and their carers are living with a great deal of uncertainty. Every client and family that we look after will react in different ways to the news that death is imminent. The reasons for this are many but include previous experiences, culture, and religious beliefs.

You will see clients and carers expressing many of the emotions you have just experienced in the above exercise. We all know that the client is an individual, but what is it that makes people different from each other? How does this affect the way that we care for them?

Caring for people who are dying is about helping to create an environment where they can feel at peace to explore the things that are important to them. It is about helping people to "live until they die", helping people to resolve relationships (goodbyes, thankyous and sorrys), and giving people the sense that they don't just have a past and present, but also a future.

Caring for the "family"

When we talk about the "family" of a client we do not necessarily mean blood relations. It is the people that the client says is closest to them. It is important to remember that sometimes the client's partner, relative or friend may wish to assist with physical care and they should be included in planning and carrying out care where this is appropriate.

Caring for the individual

Health care assistants have a key role in helping to care for people who are dying. Clients will often "open up" to those who perform essential nursing care for them. You may well find that clients confide in you. This has implications for teamwork and your own psychological support, not to mention confidentiality. It is important that clients and carers know that you are part of a team, and any confidential information given to you is kept within the team.

Nursing care

Most people who are terminally ill will spend longer periods of time at rest or in bed, and run the risk of developing pressure sores. There is often weight loss which will increase the risk. Attention to pressure areas and the provision of a specialised mattress which fits over the normal mattress can relieve some of the problems. Carers often feel that they are doing something useful if they can take part in physical care, and often like to learn how to care for clients when no one else is there.

Symptom control

We all know what it is like to feel sick, have a headache or other pain. A symptom is a physical sign from our bodies to tell us something is wrong. However, the same symptom in two different people can mean two different things. For example, a runner who is out of breath after a race knows that they have performed their "job"; for someone with advanced lung cancer it may mean that death is approaching.

Symptom control is a very important part of caring for a person who is dying. People almost always experience physical pain or discomfort when they are facing death. These physical symptoms may be associated with the illness, for example someone with a brain tumour may have headache, but there are other symptoms as well which are associated with anxiety or fear.

In addition to pain control, there are a number of specific physical problems where you can take action to help the dying person feel more comfortable in their final days.

Nausea and vomiting
Nausea and vomiting can result from the disease process itself or from medicines designed to relieve pain. It is important that anti-sickness medicines (anti-emetics) are prescribed and given regularly. These medicines need to be given before a person eats or drinks to ensure maximum effect. You should also offer mouth care or a mouthwash, and always clear up any vomiting quickly and thoroughly.

Fatigue and tiredness
Weakness and tiredness are common to many illnesses. Mutually agreed goals can be identified and set to help conserve the client's energy for important tasks that will enable them to maintain their independence. The timing and pacing of any caring activity needs to be carefully considered to allow the client time to rest and to participate in their care.

Constipation
Pain relieving medicines and lack of mobility both contribute to constipation in the client who is terminally ill. A lack of bulk in the diet and reduced intake of fluids can also affect normal bowel movement. Promoting fluid intake, providing bulk such as whole grain products in the diet and encouraging some exercise may help alleviate constipation.

Diarrhoea
Diarrhoea can result from the disease process and complications of treatment or medicines. Your approach to dealing with clients with diarrhoea is very important. Although medicines may be prescribed and a less bulky diet may be offered it is equally important for the client to be able to use any toilet facilities, commodes or bed pans as quickly as possible.

Urinary incontinence
Incontinence of urine can occur because of the disease processes or because of a reduced level of consciousness that may be caused by pain relieving medicines. Some clients may wish to have an indwelling catheter or urinary sheath. Washing and drying the skin is important to prevent irritation and barrier creams can help to make the client more comfortable.

Inadequate nutrition

Eating and drinking usually become less interesting to the client who is dying, and may be a source of great anxiety to the carer. This is because food and interest in food is often a measure of how healthy we are. Many carers get very anxious when the client is eating and drinking very little. It is important to report these kinds of worries to a qualified member of staff, and to remember that small but frequent portions of food may be better tolerated.

Enteral feeding

Enteral feeding is a system of providing liquid food through a tube that enters the stomach or small intestine directly. The tube may be inserted through the nose or surgically into the stomach. The liquid feeds may be given at regular intervals in a large syringe, or the tube may be connected to a machine that delivers the liquid feed continuously over a period of time. It is important that a qualified member of staff regularly checks the tube to ensure that it is in the correct position.

Frequent mouth care and sips of fluids or ice cubes can help clients to maintain fluid intake where they are unable to drink. This can help to alleviate thirst and enable them to feel more comfortable.

Breathing difficulties

Sitting clients in an upright position to improve their breathing capacity and to suppress coughing, can help with breathing difficulties. Suction may be available to remove secretions from the mouth and throat. If oxygen is being used it is important that it is regulated according to the care plan and that there is no smoking in the room.

Pain control

Everyone experiences pain. However, pain is highly subjective and can be dependent upon a person's emotional state, or related to cultural factors. Therefore pain assessment must always be related to the experience of the client themself and not related to how we think the severity or the place of the pain should be.

Pain assessment charts

A qualified member of staff should be able to provide "pain assessment charts". Ideally, these charts should be completed by the client themself, but there is no reason why you cannot help the person to complete the chart. Most pain assessment charts (fig 1) include a diagram and a pain scale. The diagram allows the client to indicate where on their body they are experiencing the pain. The pain scale allows them to signify how much or how severe the pain is that they are experiencing. In addition there should be space in care plans for the client to state when the pain starts, how long it lasts for and anything that aggravates the pain or sets it off.

Other indicators of pain

Some clients may not be able to tell you how they are feeling, so you should be aware of behaviour that may indicate pain. This includes sounds, such as moaning, grunting or gasping; facial expressions such as grimacing, clenched teeth or lip biting; body movement such as restlessness, increased muscle tension or hand and finger movements; and finally, avoiding conversation or having a reduced level of concentration.

As a care assistant you are in a key position to observe, monitor and report any changes in pain experienced by the client. It is important that you establish a trusting relationship so that the client feels able to tell you about any pain. Remember that this may be related to emotional feelings as well as physical pain. It is important that you ensure that pain relief is provided regularly and before the pain

Pain assessment

1. When did the pain start?

2. How long does the pain last for?

3. Where is the pain?

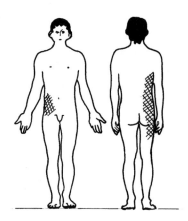

4. How severe is the pain?

1..........2..........3..........4..........5..........6..........7..........8..........9..........10
No pain   **Severe pain**

5. Does anything bring on the pain?

6. Does anything make the pain worse?

7. What helps to relieve the pain?

Other indicators:

Vocal sounds:
Moaning, crying, gasping, screaming

Facial expressions:
Grimacing, clenching teeth, wrinkled forehead, lip biting

Body movement:
Restlessness, muscle tension, reluctance to move

Social interaction:
Avoiding conversation, reduced concentration levels, focusing on pain relieving activity

Fig 1. Pain assessment chart.

becomes severe.

You can help the client to record their levels of pain and to choose pain relieving measures on the basis of their feelings and the severity of the pain that they are experiencing. Keep an open mind about what may relieve pain. Medicines may not always be required or can be supplemented by other pain controlling measures such as changing position, massaging the area, applying hot or cold compresses or ensuring that the environment is not too hot, too cold, too noisy and so on.

Syringe drivers

Clients who are terminally ill often experience chronic and persistent pain. Pain relieving medicines can be given in many different ways: tablets, liquids, suppositories and injections. In addition to these a syringe driver may also be used. This is a small battery operated pump, about the size of a portable telephone. It has a syringe filled with prescribed medication inserted into it, and delivers the medicines subcutaneously (under the skin), usually over a 24 hour period. A qualified member of staff will be responsible for setting up and monitoring the flow and rate of the infusion. You may need to observe the point at which the needle is inserted and report any swelling or redness of the area or if the pump stops and the alarm sounds.

Emotional care

People will have many different reactions when adjusting to loss through death. The most important thing for us to remember is that we are there to assist clients and their carers in coping with the uncertainty. We are often asked questions that are impossible to answer.

Difficult questions

It is important to be honest even when we do not know the answers. Pretending that the client will recover when we know they are going to die is dangerous and will quickly destroy trust when the person becomes sicker. Always admit that you do not know the answer to a difficult question. You can always ask a qualified member of staff or one of the specialist palliative care team members to see the client or their carer while you are present. This will help everyone to understand the issues that they are facing.

Anger and frustration

Sometimes clients and carers will take out their anger at their situation on us. This is because they find it too painful to express this with their loved ones. Helping to sort out these difficulties requires skill and experience in these areas and should be referred to a qualified member of staff.

Crying (including your own tears) should always be allowed to take its natural course. It is a healthy way of expressing emotional, psychological or spiritual pain. Never tell a client to cheer up. After all, they have good reason to cry.

Touching the client when they are distressed can be helpful, but be careful not to smother them. Touching the hand to show you care is much more beneficial than a big bear hug, which although tempting to do, can make the client feel you are too overbearing. However, sometimes clients may indicate to you that a hug is appropriate. Knowing these signals comes with experience.

Bereavement

Bereavement sums up the thoughts, feelings and activity that follows death and loss. It includes such things as grief and mourning. The exercise at the beginning of this chapter will help you to consider some of the issues associated with bereavement. There are many different theories on the process of bereavement and the way in which it affects people. It is part of a normal process, although you may find that you will need to continue to provide care to partners or carers long after the client that you were caring for originally has died. You may need to talk about your own experiences and feelings after the client has died and in turn you may need to offer support to those people who are left behind.

Points to remember

1. Palliative care aims to enable people to get on with living their lives in comfort, peace and without pain, while they have an illness which will ultimately end their life.

2. Specialist palliative care or support teams are available to offer support to community workers to help with practical advice for clients, their carers and staff involved in providing care to those clients who are dying.

3. Every client and family that we look after will react in different ways to the news that death is imminent. The reasons for this are many but include previous experiences, culture, and religious beliefs.

4. It is important to remember that sometimes the client's partner, relative or friend may wish to assist with the physical care of the client and they should be included in planning and carrying out care where this is appropriate.

5. Pain assessment must always be related to the experience of the client themselves and not related to how we think the severity or the place of the pain should be.

6. People will have many different reactions when adjusting to loss through death. You may experience people asking difficult questions or people showing anger and frustration.

7. Loss and bereavement is normal, but this can continue long after the client has died. Talking about your own experiences and feelings with qualified members of staff will help you to overcome any problems.

NVQ Level 2 & 3 Core Skills
O Promote equality for all individuals.
U4 Contribute to the health, safety and security of individuals and their environment.
U5 Obtain, transmit and store information relating tothe deliver of a care service.
Level 2 Core Unit
W2 Contribute to the ongoing support of clients and others significant to them.
Level 3 Core Units
Z4 Promote communication with clients where there are communication difficulties.
Z8 Support clients when they are distressed.
Y2 Enable clients to make use of available services and information.
Level 2 Direct Care
Z6 Enable clients to maintain and improve their mobility.
Z7 Contribute to the movement and treatment of clients to maximise their personal hygiene and appearance.
Z9 Enable clients to maintain their personal hygiene and appearance.
Z10 Enable clients to eat and drink.
Z11 Enable clients to access and use toilet facilities.
Z19 Enable clients to achieve physical comfort.
Level 2 Domiciliary Support
Z7 Contribute to the movement and treatment of clients to maximise their physical comfort.
W8 Enable clients to maintain contacts in potentially isolating situations.

CHAPTER 23

Carers and relatives

June Andrews and Stuart Darby

• All carers are different • Anticipating their fears • Welcome their questions, and give them answers • Make practical information available • Complaints can be a good thing • Carers support each other

Everyone needs support from other people. It can help us to cope with everyday living, particularly when we are ill or going through difficult times. The term carer is used to describe a person who looks after an elderly, disabled or sick friend or relative who cannot manage on their own at home. Most carers are women who receive no formal payment, although it is recognised that many men also care for someone at home. Carers come from all parts of society and cultures and from differing financial and environmental circumstances. The range and type of help that you can give to carers will therefore vary enormously.

All carers are different

Many carers undertake activities for dependent people that are extremely demanding. They are expected to be nurses, social workers, counsellors, look after people's finances and be housekeepers, cooks and cleaners. In addition, they usually face these tasks alone with little support physically, financially or emotionally.

Many people live alone at home. Some may have relatives who are carers and others may rely on friends or neighbours. The amount of contact with relatives will vary. Think about your own family. There may be some relatives that you only send a Christmas card to, but who live too far away to visit. On the other hand, your grandparents may live in the same town as you and be visited each day by a stream of relatives.

Some relatives may feel that they are expected to care, but for one reason or another they cannot. In addition, there are assumptions that people from Black and other ethnic minorities insist on caring for their dependent relatives, but this is not always true.

The important thing to remember is that every person is different, and their carers are different. Carers can therefore be parents, older children, partners, friends, neighbours, or someone who has been a lodger for twenty years who means more to the person than anyone else.

The way relatives respond to you, the dependent person and their caring role, may depend upon what the relationship has been like in the past:

"Mum lives alone just three miles away so we call in every day, and if the weather is good she comes out shopping with us to buy a few bits for herself."

"As I am a solicitor the family look to me to organise aunty's care and financial arrangements. Actually, my brother who is a nurse would have been a better choice but he works strange shifts and hours. She knows that she can contact me if there are any problems, but I don't see the point of going to see her – we hardly know each other anyway."

With both of these relatives you can see what the position was before a person becomes dependent and in need of help. This explains why different people take on different caring roles.

The amount of contact with carers and the type of care that they can give will also vary. For example, an older man looking after his wife may be able to shop and cook, but would feel or be physically unable to wash her or carry out intimate care.

What carers need

Anticipate their anxiety

Carers may worry you will not understand what needs to be done and they will want to ensure that they get the best possible help available. They may also worry about their own caring skills and whether they will have the physical and emotional strength to continue. They may also worry about what will happen to the dependent person if they become ill or unable to carry on caring. Carers need support and help to overcome these fears and anxieties. The following list highlights some of their needs:

Early identification of problems

Carers need to be certain that any problems that may occur will be identified early on. This will ensure that problems do not become worse or that they are prevented altogether.

Assessment

Assessing the needs of carers as well as the dependent person is important. It may include the type of help that they require and the number of hours and frequency that they need it.

Quick referrals and action

When a problem has been identified, carers need immediate help. This means referring quickly to the appropriate agency, such as the GP, physiotherapist or team for the terminally ill. Most services have a charter where they will try to respond to a referral within a given time. Imagine how you feel when you have to wait for a service engineer if your telephone is faulty?

Active medical treatment for themselves

Carers often neglect their own physical and mental health. They may be too busy looking after someone else, or hope that it will go away because they worry about the consequences of not being able to care. Encouraging carers to look after their own health will not only benefit them, but also the dependent person.

Continuity and review of services

Carers will always welcome seeing a familiar face who knows the routine and knows the dependent person. Regular review and changes to care are also needed however to ensure that it is flexible and best meets their needs.

Consultation at all levels of service planning

Carers need to be consulted about the services that are being provided and the actual care that is planned and delivered. There are many ways that you can encourage them to participate in care planning, even writing in records. This level of involvement will help to give them power and to feel in control.

Regular help with household and personal care

Regular, planned help is essential. A carer will not welcome help that "they might get sometime next week, or perhaps on Thursday morning". They need to be able to plan their lives and know that they will get support to undertake activities.

Financial support through both tax systems and benefits

Many carers are unable to earn money as their role is carried out twenty-four hours a day, seven days a week. Advice and information about financial support and all possible benefits is always welcome. Citizen's advice workers will often visit people at home. Some people may prefer to have a job, and details on respite care can help them to organise and plan this.

Provision of regular breaks, respite and long-term care

Some carers feel guilty about taking regular breaks. There are alternative types of care, such as a person attending a day hospital or day centre, as well as short periods of residential and nursing home care. This will help carers to take a break and to refresh their energies. You may also need to support carers who feel that they cannot carry on any longer, but feel guilty about seeking long-term care.

Practical information

Information and advice is always welcomed by carers. By having someone to talk to and practical advice on how to cope their lives can often be made easier. Having a commode in the bedroom for use at night, rather than having to take a person to the toilet is a simple example. What type of commode and where to get one is the type of information carers need.

It's the way you say it

The way that you tell carers about the care you are giving to a client can affect the way they feel.

You might not think that you make other people nervous, but you should consider the possibility. You are very important to carers. What you seem to think and feel

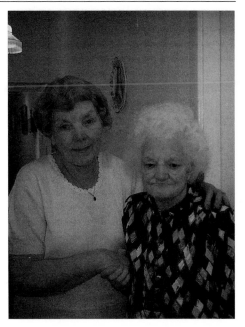

An encouraging word from you about their skills and abilities can make all the difference to a carer.

about the dependent person can make all the difference between a carer feeling good or bad about themselves or the care you give. A word from you about how a person is doing and encouragement to the carer about their skills and abilities can make them feel very much better about themselves.

But of course it can work either way. Either carers hang onto your every word and worry about all that you have said or they ignore you and ask to speak to a more senior member of staff. If you are always willing to talk, they will eventually discover that you are able to find out information for them, or the most appropriate service for further advice.

Carers will often ask the kind of question that will be covered by this book. Other questions will include general information about the service you work for, that you can answer yourself.

Remember to include carers when writing in records and to ask their opinion. You should always make sure that they know your name and how to contact your service, particularly outside office hours when the telephone number may be different.

There may be a leaflet that you can give out, or a "charter". Charters set out what services are provided, when and how they are delivered, and who is responsible for delivering them. They will usually set out the way in which a carer can contribute to shaping services, such as making suggestions for improvements and particularly how to complain.

Complaints: a good thing

There are good and bad ways of handling complaints. When carers complain they usually need at least one of three things:

• To get an explanation and an apology
• To get some compensation (not always financially)
• To draw attention to the fact that they are monitoring the quality of your service.

Most employing organisations have a formal complaints procedure. This includes a time scale by which letters or telephone complaints are dealt with. It usually includes a system for investigating complaints.

Sometimes you may take the brunt of a carer's anger. They may be tired and frustrated with caring and just need to "sound off". This is difficult to handle, particularly when you are doing your best, but a simple apology and recognition that you understand can often prevent major incidents from occurring. You should always tell the truth, but a good response includes the reason for the problem, and an indication of what is being done about it. This will often be enough to satisfy the person, but it is wise to let a more senior member of staff know about a complaint.

Getting compensation does not necessarily mean a financial payment. An increase in the number of visiting hours, visiting at different times or making greater efforts to provide more flexible care, may achieve greater satisfaction. Giving carers the opportunity to complain enables them to participate in monitoring and making changes to your service. They are the best people to decide whether a service is good or bad. Often the standards and quality of a service can be improved if carers' views are heard and acted upon.

Complaints are a good thing if they give you the chance to improve care. They also give you the chance to explain and justify the care that you give. Give carers confidence when you answer their questions. This means:

• Listen carefully to what they are saying
• Give an answer if you can
• Don't be afraid to say you don't know.
• Make sure that they know you will find someone who can give an answer.
• Make certain that a senior member of staff is aware.

Do remember that some people will feel that they cannot complain. They will be very grateful for whatever help they can get, however small. Some carers may also fear that if they complain, help will be withdrawn or reduced. This can create an added anxiety, and only by being open and honest, and encouraging them to be so too, will you provide a service that people want and that meets both your expectations and the expectations of the carer.

Change in a carer's life

Carers are often adjusting to a great change and you are making that possible. Some carers may have mixed feelings about their role, even though they love and care about the person that they look after. The caring role may have impinged upon their own role as mother or partner. They may feel that they cannot do what they want to, such as follow a career or undertake education. They may not feel able to cope with a change in role. Role reversal and conflict can occur where they are looking after a parent or partner and find that they are now the helper and the supporter.

Some carers may want to get very involved in what is happening and some will keep well out of the way. You might feel that the carer who stays away has dumped the dependent person, and doesn't care. It is useful to think about some reasons why a carer may not want to be involved in some aspects of care:

• Fear of not doing what is right and causing physical harm
• Fear of carrying out an intimate task
• Fear of upsetting you or other services and meddling
• Fear that if they do too much, you will do less or reduce your visits
• Inability to stomach certain tasks, such as caring for someone who is incontinent
• Fear of watching their loved one decline in health or die
• Fear of being left to cope without adequate help and support
• Not having the physical or mental strength to carry on.

Carers often feel very isolated, alone, and need other people to share their concerns and worries with. Talking to other people in a similar position who can understand how they feel can help tremendously.

Mutual support

When you are going through a difficult period it often helps to meet and speak to someone else with the same problem. There are practical and also emotional problems associated with caring for a person at home, and the help and advice that carers can give to each other is invaluable.

Carers groups may be started by a local authority, health or voluntary sector worker. They can also be set up by a group of like-minded carers. After a time, carers can be helped to take over groups and run them themselves. Some carers groups operate for a specific reason, such as coping with bereavement, while others may be made up of carers who also look after a person with a specific illness, such as dementia.

Carers groups have many functions: the chance to share experiences and provide mutual support is the commonest. Other groups will provide practical help and information as well. An added bonus of most carers groups is the opportunity for friendship and social activities to take place. This takes them away from caring and gives them a chance to look after and think about themselves, rather than someone else.

Coping with death
When a client dies you will have a mixture of feelings to deal with. You may feel sorrow and loss, but also happy that you were able to make their last hours comfortable. You will also have to deal with the feelings of carers and family.

It is said that when a person becomes terminally ill, and perhaps confused or unable to look after themselves, part of their personality dies. A daughter may say, "That's not my mother talking. She must be feeling awful that we have to do so much for her and she cannot be independent". Carers will often say that it is as if they are already dead. The real person that they know and love has just left, and the body left behind is just a shadow of the real person.

So when that person eventually dies, it is a second death for the carer. They may say that they feel better that the person is dead or that they feel relieved because now they can mourn, although the person died some time before when they became very ill. Some people may be very distressed if they were not present when a person died. The death may have been sudden and unexpected so the carer may have the shock of visiting or receiving a telephone call or message out of the blue.

Showing as much respect to the carer as you did for the client is an important part of providing support and help. You may wish to sit with the carer just talking through what has happened and shedding some tears. Helping carers with their last duties can be sad, but satisfying. You know that you have done your best and you can therefore understand how a carer will feel. They don't just lose the person that they cared for, but also all the friendships and people they may have met in the course of their caring role.

This is why many services will continue to visit a carer long after a client has died. (And many carers stay involved in the carers group, with the friends they have made.) The experience of bereavement is something that can be shared with others. You may also appreciate the chance to talk to a carer, to express your own condolences, and to continue to provide support and advice where appropriate.

Points to remember

1. All carers will be different, so their involvement will be different.
2. Carers may be anxious, and you can help them by anticipating their fears.
3. If you welcome questions and help to find answers it will make them less anxious.
4. You can ensure practical information is available to them.
5. The way you tell carers about the care you are giving to a client can affect the way they feel.
6. Complaints can be a good thing if handled sensitively.
7. Carers are often adjusting to a great change and you are making that possible.
8. Carers often get support from each other.

Further reading

Nancy Korner (1988) – *Caring at home. A Handbook for people looking after someone young or old, handicapped or disabled, ill or frail.* National Extension College.

NVQ Levels 2 & 3 Core Units

O Promote equality for all individuals.
U4 Contribute to the health, safety and security of individuals and their environment.
U5 Obtain, transmit and store information relating to the delivery of a care service.

Level 2 Core Unit

W2 Contribute to the ongoing support of clients and others significant to them.

Level 3 Core Units

Z8 Support clients when they are distressed.
Y2 Enable clients to make use of available services and information.

Level 2 Domiciliary support

Y1 Enable clients to manage their domestic and personal resources.
W8 Enable clients to maintain contacts in potentially isolating situations.
U1 Contribute to the maintenance and management of domestic and personal resources.

CHAPTER 24

National Vocational Qualifications

by Judith Roberts

What are NVQs and what use are they to you? • The way training and assessment works • How you can get started

National Vocational Qualifications (NVQs) are a country wide system of qualifications related to job skills and occupations. In Scotland they are called Scottish Vocational Qualifications (SVQs). NVQs/SVQs apply not only to the care sector, but are also available in many other fields of work, from horse grooming to hairdressing, motor vehicle repair to management.

All NVQ awards are based on the idea of competence – the ability to perform in the workplace, to the standards that the occupation requires.

An NVQ is gained when the candidate is assessed performing in a real work situation, doing a real job, to the required standards. But skills on their own are not enough. The worker has to show that they understand why they are doing the task in

The benefits of NVQs

• NVQs allow you to build up parts of the award, or "credits", gradually. It doesn't matter when you do them or how long it takes. This helps people fit in training around domestic or work commitments.

• There is open access: anyone can apply to be assessed.

• Assessment can be obtained and achieved independently of the time or methods of any accompanying learning. Distance or Open Learning becomes a practical solution for people who work unsocial hours.

• NVQs do not demand time away from the workplace, and their development and the assessment process is directly relevant and meaningful to the worker.

• It is learning by doing, an active process that for many people makes the learning process more enjoyable, more relevant and more effective.

Why get involved?

Candidates who have achieved NVQ awards in Care have said that the process of becoming qualified has meant:

• They are more aware of their clients' needs and rights, especially their emotional, social and cultural needs.

• They feel they now give more individualised care, and are more useful to other members of the team.

• They are now more aware of the "How?" and "Why?" of their practice, and are able to describe their experience using a more "professional" vocabulary.

• They consider themselves to be better informed, more assertive and confident, and better able to challenge inadequate practice.

• They found the support and recognition offered to them by their work based assessor valuable, and often developed more effective working relations with others.

that way; in other words some "under-pinning knowledge" is necessary.

Standards have been decided on, after years of work developing and testing them, by representatives from each field of work, called Lead Industry Bodies (LIB). The LIB for the care sector is the Care Sector Consortium.

NVQs are awarded by organisations called Awarding Bodies. Examples are City and Guilds, the Central Council for Education and Training in Social Work (CCETSW), and BTEC.

Levels of awards

All NVQs are graded, rising from Level 1 to Level 5. The higher the level, the greater the breadth and complexity of the qualification. This allows the worker to progress within the qualification structure as their skills, knowledge and responsibilities increase and broaden.

Level 1 Foundation/ basic work activities
Level 2 A broad range of skills and responsibilities
Level 3 Complex/skilled and/or supervisory work
Level 4 Managerial/specialist
Level 5 Professional/senior managerial

The NVQ framework

NVQ awards have a common structure. Each different **level** is made up of a number of **units**. These units are in turn split into several **elements** of competence.

Each element contains **performance criteria** (details of what is expected of you as you perform the task), **range statements** where you need to show competence in a range of care situations, and details of the **underpinning knowledge** you are required to show.

Taking one **element** at a time, the worker is assessed working in each of the situations specified in the element. Their standard of competence is assessed against the **performance criteria** and **underpin-**

ning knowledge that element requires. Through this process the worker can slowly build up their qualification. This is called "credit accumulation".

NVQs Awards in Care:
the Integrated Standards

NVQs in both social care and nursing settings have been brought together, and there are qualifications available at Levels 2 and 3. These awards give care workers more choice and opportunity for progression in jobs across both sectors, and represent more closely the wide range of client groups, roles and responsibilities.

To the structure of units and elements described before, **endorsements** are added. These are units grouped together because they relate to the specific role of the candidate. In addition there is **Unit O – Promote equality for all individuals –** that is assessed during every assessment.

For example, care assistants working with elderly people need some of the same skills and knowledge, and some different skills and knowledge, from care assistants working in postnatal departments. So both will work through the same Core Units as described earlier, plus the Endorsement for their work area.

People involved in the assessment process

A *candidate* is the worker being assessed for an NVQ.

An *assessor* is the person who carries out the assessment of the candidate. The assessor is usually a more senior colleague who has a broad expertise in the work. Increasingly it is expected that the assessor will also have proved they are competent to assess the work of others.

The assessor's decisions are checked by a person called the *Internal Verifier* (IV) whose role is to make sure that the assessments carried out by the assessor meet the NVQ standards and the Awarding Body assessment requirements. This per-

How to start

There are three main processes involved:

1. Collect information so that you can see which Levels and Endorsements would be best for you.

2. Identify your training requirements and how you can obtain any necessary training.

3. Find out how, and by whom, you can be assessed in the workplace. It is possible that your employer is already associated with an assessment centre.

Remember, without the opportunity for assessment, and verification of the assessment, you will not get your qualification.

1. Information gathering

You will need to find out:

• Is your workplace considering getting involved with NVQs? Whom should you contact, where and when? This is not always easy if you work nights or weekends, but persevere. It is likely that other care assistants, the matron or manager will know more.

• More information about NVQs, and especially about NVQs in Care. This information should be available from your training department, but it also could be obtained from the Career Service, the local Training and Enterprise Council (TEC), the National Council for Vocational Qualifications, your union or local colleges, or the awarding body. The UK Central Council for Nursing and Midwifery has decided that possession of a Level 3 Care NVQ could be a possible entry qualification into Nurse Education – but it is **not** automatic. Each school of Health may have additional requirements.

• Which level of award and choice of endorsement would be appropriate for you? This will be decided in discussion with your immediate line manager and the training centre.

• What existing knowledge could you be accredited with, and what additional training might you require?

• When are you likely to be accepted onto an NVQ programme and offered assessment? There may be some delay, so it could be useful to see if there are any appropriate programmes or short courses you could attend while waiting. Accreditation of Prior Learning should be available, so this would not be wasted.

• What costs, if any, might you have to pay towards your assessment? Ask whether your local TEC is sponsoring NVQs, especially if there is any financial support.

• Where will any training occur? Will you have to do it in your own time? Is attendance at the training sessions compulsory?

• How quickly will they expect you to complete all your assessments? (Less than six months is unrealistic unless you and your assessor are very committed and your establishment not too busy.)

• Is there open access? Do you have to be employed for a certain length of time? Will they only assess day staff? (They shouldn't – this could contravene their equal opportunities policy.)

• Do you have to be recommended by your line manager?

• Will they expect you to stay in employment for a stated length of time following completion – or pay any fees back?

• Will you be allowed to progress to Level 3? This will depend upon your role – you cannot do a Level 3 qualification unless you are doing the relevant work, as you would not be able to be assessed otherwise.

2. Undertake any training or development required

This could be through a variety of routes and take varying lengths of time. It is recommended that for a Level 2 award training should take between six and ten months, and for a Level 3 award about one year. Obviously it depends on your previous knowledge, and how recently any training took place. This handbook would be a very useful resource for your training. When enquiring about your training, find answers to the following questions:

• Does your workplace offer training on site or do you have to go elsewhere for it?

• How many actual hours of tuition will you receive? How big are the classes?

• Is there access to a library? Are any other resources available?

• What methods will be used to deliver the "underpinning knowledge"? Will any specialists be teaching you? How much tutorial support will you be offered?

3. Getting assessed in the workplace
This will depend upon the policy of your employer. You should be able to find out who is to be your assesssor, so make time to get to know them (although it will probably be someone you have already worked with).

Don't forget that at first both you and your assessor may be anxious or uncertain. You may have to develop a working relationship that suits you both.

The "Standards" may look like a foreign language, but after time and lots of reading they do become more "user-friendly". So once you are given the Standards, do start to read them. Ask if you do not understand a word or phrase – others are probably wondering too!

Start taking notice of your practice and the practice of others, reflect on what you observe and discuss it if you can with your assessor or tutor. Trust yourself: you may have things to learn, but don't forget you are already doing the job. You probably know more than you think.

son may come from a different work setting or section from the assessor.

Finally the work of the Internal Verifier is checked by an *External Verifier*, who is appointed by the Awarding Body and has no connection with your workplace.

Your assessment

The assessment methods are designed to be flexible and easily organised, with the assessment timetable being devised and controlled by the candidate. This is called "Assessment on demand".

The commonest method of assessment, particularly in care, is assessment by direct observation of the candidate's work. However, another eight methods are also acceptable, These can include simulations (role playing), oral or written questions, assignments, completion of work products such as reports or records, testimony of others (clients, other workers), or the candidate's explanation of the process or review of work. These other assessment methods are particularly useful when candidates do not regularly work with their assessor.

However, often for NVQ Level 2 Care Awards, direct observation is the most practical. A typical assessment might run as follows:

1 A worker checks the assessment requirements of the element. They check to see if they have sufficient underpinning knowledge and skills. They may ask the opinion of an impartial adviser to help decide this. They may decide to undertake training or support. The training could be "in house", from a more senior colleague or training officer, or from a planned programme.

2 Following training the candidate checks that they now have the required knowledge and skills, and they are ready for assessment.

3 The candidate approaches their assessor, and requests assessment. The assessor talks about the impending assessment, checks the candidate is fully aware of the assessment requirements, and might offer to do a "practice assessment". They will discuss any queries, and only when they *both* feel confident that the worker is ready to be assessed will they arrange a date that suits them both.

In the case of the care awards, they also approach a suitable client or clients, to ask if they would agree to be involved. It is vitally important that the client gives informed consent, and is not coerced in any way. If a client is confused or has limited understanding, the family should be asked for permission if at all possible.

4 The assessment day. The candidate will confirm with the client that they are still happy to be involved and the assessor will confirm that the candidate is ready. Throughout whatever activity is taking place the assessor will observe the candidate, as unobtrusively as possible.

After the observation of the candidate's practice the assessor will question the candidate, and may ask to see any relevant documentation or reports. This helps the assessor to check on any aspects of the assessment process and helps to make sure that the candidate has the understanding and knowledge specified in the standards. Then, and only then, will the assessor confirm to the candidate their decision: either the candidate is competent or not yet competent.

Once the decision has been recorded, the assessor will explain to the candidate, in as much detail as is required, why they made that decision, if necessary giving comments or advice that will help the candidate improve their future practice.

At the end of the process they will make an appointment for the assessment of a new element, or if necessary a re-assessment. All necessary documentation is completed and made available for the Internal Verifier to see.

5 Once the assessor has completed a few assessments the IV will be invited to check on the documentation and the candidates' records of evidence.

6 Finally when all the units of the award have been assessed and the candidate is declared competent, the External Verifier will be invited to visit the assessment centre to view the assessment records (probably those of other candidates as well). They will make their decision based upon the evidence they check. Once the assessments have External Verifier approval the candidates will receive their qualification certificates.

See page 187 for useful addresses.

Awards in Care
NVQs/SVQs Level 2

Level 2 Core

O Promote equality for all individuals

Z1 Contribute to the protection of individuals from abuse

W2 Contribute to the ongoing support of clients and others significant to them

W3 Support clients in transition due to their care requirements

U4 Contribute to the health, safety and security of individuals and their environment

U5 Obtain, transmit and store information relating to the delivery of a care service

Direct Care Endorsement

Z6 Enable clients to maintain and improve their mobility

Z7 Contribute to the movement and treatment of clients to maximise their physical comfort

Z9 Enable clients to maintain their personal hygiene and appearance

Z10 Enable clients to eat and drink

Z11 Enable clients to access and use toilet facilities

Z19 Enable clients to achieve physical comfort

These are the Units you need to work through to achieve NVQ Level 2 in Care with the Direct Care Endorsement.

NVQ Subject Index

This chart shows the Units of National Vocational Qualification Awards in Care which are covered (partly or completely) in the chapters of this book.

	Ch 1	Ch 2	Ch 3	Ch 4	Ch 5	Ch 6	Ch 7	Ch 8	Ch 9	Ch 10	Ch 11	Ch 12	Ch 13	Ch 14	Ch 15	Ch 16	Ch 17	Ch 18	Ch 19	Ch 20	Ch 21	Ch 22	Ch 23
Level II Core																							
O	•	•	•	•	•	•	•		•	•	•	•	•	•	•	•	•		•	•	•	•	•
Z 1		•	•								•	•			•					•	•		
W 2	•	•	•	•	•	•	•	•		•	•	•	•	•	•	•	•	•	•	•	•	•	
W 3						•									•								
U 4	•	•	•	•	•	•	•	•	•	•	•	•	•	•	•	•	•	•	•	•	•	•	•
U 5	•	•	•	•	•	•	•	•	•	•	•	•	•	•	•	•	•	•	•	•	•	•	•
Developmental Care																							
Z 5					•				•						•		•						
Z 13	•				•	•	•	•	•				•		•	•							•
X 1									•			•			•								
W 8			•	•	•	•	•		•	•		•	•		•	•				•	•	•	•
U 2						•			•						•	•	•	•	•			•	
Direct Care																							
Z 6				•					•	•			•		•	•	•	•				•	
Z 7									•						•	•	•					•	
Z 9					•				•						•	•	•	•				•	
Z 10			•		•	•			•						•	•						•	
Z 11			•		•	•			•						•	•		•				•	
Z 19					•				•						•	•		•				•	
Domiciliary Support																							
Z 7									•						•	•	•					•	
Y 1		•									•		•		•								•
W 8	•		•	•	•	•	•		•			•	•		•	•				•	•	•	•
U 1		•			•				•				•		•				•				•
Special Care																							
Z 9									•						•	•	•					•	
Z 10			•		•	•			•						•	•						•	
Z 13	•				•	•	•	•	•				•		•	•							•
Y 1		•									•		•		•								•
X 1									•			•			•								
W 8			•	•	•	•	•		•			•	•		•	•				•	•	•	•

184

Level III Core

	Ch 1	Ch 2	Ch 3	Ch 4	Ch 5	Ch 6	Ch 7	Ch 8	Ch 9	Ch 10	Ch 11	Ch 12	Ch 13	Ch 14	Ch 15	Ch 16	Ch 17	Ch 18	Ch 19	Ch 20	Ch 21	Ch 22	Ch 23
O	•	•	•	•	•	•	•	•	•	•	•	•	•	•	•	•	•	•	•	•	•	•	•
Z 1			•								•	•							•	•	•		
Z 3													•							•	•		
Z 4			•	•	•	•			•	•			•		•					•	•	•	
Z 8					•		•			•		•			•	•				•	•	•	•
Y 2	•	•	•	•	•	•	•	•	•	•	•	•	•	•	•	•	•	•	•	•	•	•	•
U 4	•	•	•	•	•	•	•	•	•	•	•	•	•	•	•	•	•	•	•	•	•	•	•
U 5	•	•	•	•	•	•	•	•	•	•	•	•	•	•	•	•	•	•	•	•	•	•	•

Promoting Independence

	Ch 1	Ch 2	Ch 3	Ch 4	Ch 5	Ch 6	Ch 7	Ch 8	Ch 9	Ch 10	Ch 11	Ch 12	Ch 13	Ch 14	Ch 15	Ch 16	Ch 17	Ch 18	Ch 19	Ch 20	Ch 21	Ch 22	Ch 23
Z 2	•	•	•	•	•	•	•	•	•	•	•	•	•	•	•	•	•	•	•	•	•	•	•
Y 3		•																					
Y 5	•										•	•			•				•			•	
X 2							•			•		•							•				
W 5			•									•	•		•	•				•	•	•	•
V 2	•	•	•	•	•	•	•	•	•	•	•	•	•	•	•	•	•	•	•	•	•	•	•

Supported Living

	Ch 1	Ch 2	Ch 3	Ch 4	Ch 5	Ch 6	Ch 7	Ch 8	Ch 9	Ch 10	Ch 11	Ch 12	Ch 13	Ch 14	Ch 15	Ch 16	Ch 17	Ch 18	Ch 19	Ch 20	Ch 21	Ch 22	Ch 23
Z 18																				•	•		
X 2							•			•		•							•				
W 1	•	•	•	•	•	•	•	•	•	•	•	•	•	•	•	•	•	•	•	•	•	•	•
W 5			•									•	•		•	•				•	•	•	•
V 2	•	•	•	•	•	•	•	•	•	•	•	•	•	•	•	•	•	•	•	•	•	•	•

Rehabilitation

	Ch 1	Ch 2	Ch 3	Ch 4	Ch 5	Ch 6	Ch 7	Ch 8	Ch 9	Ch 10	Ch 11	Ch 12	Ch 13	Ch 14	Ch 15	Ch 16	Ch 17	Ch 18	Ch 19	Ch 20	Ch 21	Ch 22	Ch 23
Y 4	•	•	•	•	•	•	•	•	•	•	•	•	•	•	•	•	•	•	•	•	•	•	•
X 2							•			•		•							•				
X 16												•											
W 1	•	•	•	•	•	•	•	•	•	•	•	•	•	•	•	•	•	•	•	•	•	•	•
W 5			•									•	•		•	•				•	•	•	•
V 1	•	•	•	•	•	•	•	•	•	•	•	•	•	•	•	•	•	•	•	•	•	•	•

Continuing Care

	Ch 1	Ch 2	Ch 3	Ch 4	Ch 5	Ch 6	Ch 7	Ch 8	Ch 9	Ch 10	Ch 11	Ch 12	Ch 13	Ch 14	Ch 15	Ch 16	Ch 17	Ch 18	Ch 19	Ch 20	Ch 21	Ch 22	Ch 23
Z 12									•	•			•		•	•	•	•	•			•	
Y 4	•	•	•	•	•	•	•	•	•	•	•	•	•	•	•	•	•	•	•	•	•	•	•
X 2							•			•		•							•				
Z 13	•				•	•	•	•					•			•	•						•
X 16												•											
V 1	•	•	•	•	•	•	•	•	•	•	•	•	•	•	•	•	•	•	•	•	•	•	•

185

	Ch 1	Ch 2	Ch 3	Ch 4	Ch 5	Ch 6	Ch 7	Ch 8	Ch 9	Ch 10	Ch 11	Ch 12	Ch 13	Ch 14	Ch 15	Ch 16	Ch 17	Ch 18	Ch 19	Ch 20	Ch 21	Ch 22	Ch 23

Supportive Long Term Care

	Ch 1	Ch 2	Ch 3	Ch 4	Ch 5	Ch 6	Ch 7	Ch 8	Ch 9	Ch 10	Ch 11	Ch 12	Ch 13	Ch 14	Ch 15	Ch 16	Ch 17	Ch 18	Ch 19	Ch 20	Ch 21	Ch 22	Ch 23
Z 12									•	•			•		•	•	•	•	•			•	
Z 10			•		•	•			•						•	•						•	
X 12			•			•	•	•	•					•	•	•	•	•	•			•	
Z 13	•					•	•	•	•				•		•	•							•
V 1	•	•	•	•	•	•	•	•	•	•	•	•	•	•	•	•	•	•	•	•	•	•	•
U 3								•		•						•			•				

Terminal Care

	Ch 1	Ch 2	Ch 3	Ch 4	Ch 5	Ch 6	Ch 7	Ch 8	Ch 9	Ch 10	Ch 11	Ch 12	Ch 13	Ch 14	Ch 15	Ch 16	Ch 17	Ch 18	Ch 19	Ch 20	Ch 21	Ch 22	Ch 23
Z 6				•					•	•			•		•	•	•	•				•	
Z 14															•	•						•	
Z 15															•							•	
X 13															•	•			•			•	
U 3								•		•						•			•				

Acute Care - Children

	Ch 1	Ch 2	Ch 3	Ch 4	Ch 5	Ch 6	Ch 7	Ch 8	Ch 9	Ch 10	Ch 11	Ch 12	Ch 13	Ch 14	Ch 15	Ch 16	Ch 17	Ch 18	Ch 19	Ch 20	Ch 21	Ch 22	Ch 23
Z 20									•														
X 12									•														
X 19																							
W 7									•														
U 3									•		•					•			•				

Support & Protection

	Ch 1	Ch 2	Ch 3	Ch 4	Ch 5	Ch 6	Ch 7	Ch 8	Ch 9	Ch 10	Ch 11	Ch 12	Ch 13	Ch 14	Ch 15	Ch 16	Ch 17	Ch 18	Ch 19	Ch 20	Ch 21	Ch 22	Ch 23
Z 2	•	•	•	•	•	•	•	•	•	•	•	•	•	•	•	•	•	•	•	•	•	•	•
Z 18																				•	•		
Y 4	•	•	•	•	•	•	•	•	•	•	•	•	•	•	•	•	•	•	•	•	•	•	•
X 2						•				•		•							•				
W 5			•									•	•		•	•			•	•	•	•	•
V 1	•	•	•	•	•	•	•	•	•	•	•	•	•	•	•	•	•	•	•	•	•	•	•

Mental Health Care

	Ch 1	Ch 2	Ch 3	Ch 4	Ch 5	Ch 6	Ch 7	Ch 8	Ch 9	Ch 10	Ch 11	Ch 12	Ch 13	Ch 14	Ch 15	Ch 16	Ch 17	Ch 18	Ch 19	Ch 20	Ch 21	Ch 22	Ch 23
Z 2	•	•	•	•	•	•	•	•	•	•	•	•	•	•	•	•	•	•	•	•	•	•	•
X 2						•				•		•							•				
X 16												•											
W 1	•	•	•	•	•	•	•	•	•	•	•	•	•	•	•	•	•	•	•	•	•	•	•
W 5	•			•			•	•			•	•			•	•			•	•	•	•	•
W 8			•	•	•	•	•		•	•		•	•		•	•			•	•	•	•	

Mobility & Movement

	Ch 1	Ch 2	Ch 3	Ch 4	Ch 5	Ch 6	Ch 7	Ch 8	Ch 9	Ch 10	Ch 11	Ch 12	Ch 13	Ch 14	Ch 15	Ch 16	Ch 17	Ch 18	Ch 19	Ch 20	Ch 21	Ch 22	Ch 23
Z 7									•						•	•	•					•	
X 9									•														
U 2							•		•						•	•	•	•	•			•	

Useful addresses

All these organisations welcome a stamped, self-addressed envelope sent with your enquiry.

Action for Dysphasic Adults, Canterbury House, 1 Royal Street, London SE1 7LN. Tel: 071 261 9572.

Action for Sick Children, Argyle House 29-31 Euston Road, London NW1 2SD. Tel: 071 833 2041.

Action for Victims of Medical Accidents, Bank Chambers, 1 London Road, Forest Hill, London SE23 3TP. Tel: 081 291 2793.

Action on Elder Abuse, Age Concern England, Astral House, 1268 London Road London SW16 4ER. Tel: 081 679 8000.

Action on Smoking and Health (ASH), 109, Gloucester Place, London. W1H 3IH. Tel: 071 935 3519.

Afro Caribbean Mental Health Association, 35-37 Electric Avenue, Brixton, London SW9 8JP. 071 737 3603.

Afro Caribbean Society for the Blind, 12 Lilac Gardens, Shirley, Surrey CR0 8NR.

Age Concern England, Astral House, 1268 London Road, London SW16 4ER. Tel: 081 679 8000.

Age Exchange Reminiscence Centre, 11 Blackheath Village, London SE3 9LA. Tel: 081 318 9105.

AIDS Helpline, National. Tel: 0800 567 123. Ethnic minority language lines also available.

Alcoholics Anonymous (AA), PO Box 1 Stonebow House, Stonebow, York. YO1 2NJ.

Alcohol Concern, 275 Grays Inn Road, London WC1. Tel: 071 833 3471.

Alzheimer's Disease Society, Gordon House, 10 Greencoat Place London SW1P 1PH. Tel: 071 306 0606.

Arthritis and Rheumatism Council (ARC), Copeman House, St Mary's Court, St Mary's Gate Chesterfield Derbyshire S41 7TD. Tel: 0246 558033.

Arthritis Care, 5 Grosvenor Crescent, London SW1X 7ER. Tel: 071 235 0902.

ASBAH (Association for Spina Bifida and Hydrocephalus), Asbah House, 42 Park Road, Peterborough PE1 2UQ. Tel: 0733 555988.

Asian People's Disability Alliance, Ground Floor, Willesden Hospital, Harlesden Rd, London NW10. Tel: 081 459 5793.

Association for all Speech Impaired Children (AFASIC), 347 Central Markets, Smithfield, London EC1A 9NH. Tel: 071 236 3632.

Association for Continence Advice, 2 Doughty Street, London WC1N 2PH. Tel: 071 404 6821.

Association of Blind Asians, 322 Upper St, London N1 2XQ. Tel: 071 226 1950.

Association of Continence Advisers, at the Disabled Living Foundation, 380-384 Harrow Road, London W9 2HU. Tel: 071 289 6111.

Association of Crossroads Care Attendant Schemes Ltd, 10 Regents Place Rugby, Warwickshire. CV21 2PN. Tel: 078 573653.

Black HIV & AIDS Network, 11 Devonport Rd., London, W12 8PB

or: 1st Floor, St Stephen's House, 41 Uxbridge Road, London W12 8LH Tel: 081 749 2828.

Breast Care and Mastectomy Association of Great Britain, 15-19 Britten St, London SW3 3TZ. 071 867 8275. Helpline 071 867 1103.

British Association of Cancer United Patients BACUP), 3 Bath Place, London EC2A 3JR. Tel.: 071 696 9003.

British Association of the Hard of Hearing, 7-11 Armstrong Road, London W3 7JL. Tel: 081 743 1110.

British Association of Occupational Therapists, 6-8 Marshalsea Rd, Southwark, London SE1 1HL. Tel: 071 357 6480.

British Colostomy Association, 38-39 Eccleston Square, London SW1V 1PB. Tel: 071 828 5175.

British Complementary Medicine Association, Exmoor Street, London W10 6DZ. Tel: 081 964 1205.

British Deaf Association, 38 Victoria Place, Carlisle. Tel: 0228 48844.

British Dental Health Foundation, Eastlands Court, St Peters Road, Warwickshire CV21 3QP. Tel: 07788 546365.

British Diabetic Association, 10 Queen Anne Street, London W1M 0BD. 071 323 1531.

British Digestive Foundation, 3 St Andrews Place Regents Park London NW1 4LB. Tel: 071 487 5332.

British Epilepsy Association, Anstey House, 40 Hanover Square, Leeds LS3 1BE. Tel: 0532 439393. (local call charge only).

British Heart Foundation, 14 Fitzhardinge St, London W1H 4DH. Tel: 071 935 0185.

British Institute of Learning Disabilities, Information and Resource Centre, Wolverhampton Rd, Kidderminster, Worcs DY10 3PP. Tel: 0562 850251.

British Kidney Patient Association, Bordon, Hampshire GU35 9JZ. Tel: 0420 472 021/2.

British Pregnancy Advisory Service, Austy Manor, Wootton Wawen, Solihull, West Midlands B95 6BX. Tel: 0564 793225.

British Red Cross Society, 9 Grosvenor Crescent, London SW1X 7EJ. Tel: 071 235 5454. Volunteer beauty care and other services.

Brittle Bone Society, 112 City Road, Dundee DD2 2PW. Tel: 0382 67603.

BTEC (Business and Technology Education Council), Central House, Upper Woburn Place, London WC1H 0HH. Tel: 071 413 8400.

Cancer Care Society, 21 Zetland Rd, Redland, Bristol BS6 7AH. Tel: 0272 427 419/232302.

Cancer Relief Macmillan Fund, 15-19 Britten St, London SW3 3TZ. Tel: 071 351 7811.

Carers National Association, 29 Chilworth Mews, London W2 3RG. Tel: 071 724 7776.

Central Council for Education and Training in Social Work (CCETSW), Derbyshire House, St Chad Street, London WC1H 8AD. Tel: 071 278 2455.

Centre for Policy on Ageing, 25-31 Ironmonger Row, London EC1V 3QP. Tel: 071 253 1787.

Chartered Society of Physiotherapy, 14 Bedford Row, London WC1. Tel: 071 242 1941.

Chest, Heart and Stroke Association, CHSA House, 123-127 Whitecross St, London EC1Y 8JJ. Tel: 071 490 7999.

Child Growth Foundation (CGF), 2, Mayfield Avenue, Chiswick, London W4 1PW. Tel: 081 995 0257.

Child Poverty Action Group (CPAG), 1-5 Bath Street, London. C1V 9PY. Tel: 071 265 3406.

Chinese Mental Health Association, c/o Working World Trust, Unit 20, Peterley Business Centre, 472 Hackney Road, London E2 9EQ. 071 613 1008.

Christian Council on Ageing, Mrs Margaret Young, 24 Cornwall Road, Harrogate, N. Yorks. HG1 2PP. Tel/Fax: 0423 504 380.

City and Guilds, 46 Brittania Street, London WC1X 9RG. Tel: 071 278 2468.

Citizens Advice Bureau, (National Association of) Myddleton House, 115-123 Pentonville Road, London, N1 9LZ. Tel: 071 833 2181.

Cleft Lip and Palate Association (CLAPA), 1, Eastwood Gardens, Kenton, Newcastle-upon-Tyne. NE3 3DQ. Tel: 091 285 9396.

College of Speech and Language Therapists, Lechmere Rd, London NW2 5BU. Tel: 071 613 3855.

Commission for Racial Equality, Eliot House, Allington St, London SW1. Tel: 071 828 7022.

Community Health Councils for England and Wales, (Association of), 30, Drayton Park, London N5 1PB. Tel: 071 609 8485

Counsel and Care for the Elderly, Twyman House, 16 Bonny Street, London NW1 9PG. Tel: 071 485 1550.

Cruse – Bereavement Care, Cruse House, 126 Sheen Road, Richmond, Surrey TW9 1UR. Tel: 081 940 4818.

Cystic Fibrosis Trust, Alexandra House, 5

Blythe Rd, Bromley, Kent BR1 3RS. Tel: 081 464 7211.

Department of Health, Richmond House, 79 Whitehall, London SW1A 2NS. Tel: 071 210 3000.

Disability Alliance Educational and Research Association, 1st Floor East, Universal House, Wentworth Street. London E1 7SA. Tel: 071 247 8776.

Disabled Living Foundation, 380-384 Harrow Road, London W9 2HU. Tel: 071 289 6111.

Down's Syndrome Association, 155 Mitcham Rd, London SW17 9PG. Tel: 081 682 4001.

District Nursing Association, 3 Albermarle Way, London. EC1V 4JB. Tel: 0903 245941.

Dyslexia Association.

Dyslexia Association (British), 98, London Road, Reading Berkshire. RG1 5AU. Tel: 0734 668271.

Endometriosis Society, 35 Belgrave Square, London SW1 8PQ. Tel: 071 235 4136/7.

English National Board for Nursing, Midwifery and Health Visiting, Victory House, Tottenham Court Road, London. W1P 0HA. Tel: 071 388 3131.

Equal Opportunities Commission, Overseas House, Quay St, Manchester M3 3HN. Tel: 061 833 9244.

ERIC: Enuresis Resource Information Centre, 65, St Michael's Hill Bristol BS2 8DZ. Tel: 0272 264920. Provides information on day and night-time wetting.

Eczema National Society, 4 Tavistock Place, London WC1H 9RA. Tel: 071 399 4097.

Family Planning Association, 27-35 Morimer Street, London, W1N 7RJ. Tel: 071 636 7866.

Friedreich's Ataxia Group, Copse Edge, Thursley Rd, Elstead, Godalming, Surrey GU8 6DJ. Tel: 0252 702 864.

Haemophilia Society, 123 Westminster Bridge Road, London SE1 7HR. Tel: 071 928 2020.

Headway (National Head Injuries Association Ltd) King Edward Court, 7 King Edward St, Nottingham. Tel: 0602 240800.

Health and Safety Executive (HSE), Broad Lane, Sheffield, S3 7HQ. Tel: 0742 89245.

Health Education Authority, Hamilton House, Mabledon Place, London. WC1H 9TX. Tel: 071 383 3833.

Health Visitors Association, 50, Southwark Street, London SE1 7HQ. Tel: 0742 892345.

Help the Aged, 16-18 St James's Walk, Clerkenwell, London EC1R 0BE. Tel: 071 253 0253.

Hospice Information Service, St Christophers Hospice, 51-59 Lawrie Park Road, Sydenham, London, SE26 6DZ. Tel: 081 778 9252.

Housing Advice Switchboard, 7A/B Fortess Road London NW5 1AD. Tel: 071 434 2522.

Huntingdon's Disease (Association to Combat), 108 Battersea High St, London SW11 3HP. Tel: 071 223 7000.

Hysterectomy Support Network, 3 Lynne Close, Green Street Green, Orpington, Kent BR6 6BS.

Ileostomy Association, PO Box 23, Mansfield, Notts NG18 4TT. Tel: 0623 28099.

Jewish Care, Stewart Young House, 221 Golders Green Road, London NW11 9DQ. Tel: 081 458 3282.

Kings Fund Centre, 126, Albert Street, London NW1 7NF. Tel: 071 267 6111.

Laryngectomy Clubs (National Association), Ground Floor, 6 Rickett St, Fulham, London SW6 1RU. Tel: 071 381 9993.

Limbless Association, 31 The Mall, Ealing, London W5 2PX. Tel: 081 579 1758.

Marie Curie Cancer Care, 28 Belgrave Square, London SW1X 8QG. Tel: 071 235 3325.

Medic Alert Foundation, 12 Bridge Wharf, 156, Caledonian Road, London. N1 9UU. Tel: 071 833 3034.

MENCAP, Royal Society for Mentally Handicapped Children and Adults, 123 Golden Lane, London EC1Y 0RT. Tel: 071 454 0454.

Mental Health Foundation, 8 Hallam Street, London W1N 6DH.

MIND/National Association for Mental Health, Granta House, 15-19 Broadway, Stratford E15 4BO. Tel: 081 519 2122.

Mobility Information Service, National Mobility Centre, Unit 2a. Atcham Industrial Estate, Shrewsbury SY4 4UG. Tel: 0743 761 889.

Motability, Gate House, West Gate, Harlow, Essex. CM20 1HR. Tel: 0279 635666.

Motor Neurone Disease Association, PO Box 246, Northampton NN1 2PR. Tel: 0604 22269/250505. Helpline 0345 626262.

Multiple Sclerosis Society of Great Britain and Northern Ireland, 25 Effie Road, Fulham, London SW6 1EE. Tel: 071 736 6267.

Muscular Dystrophy Group, 7-11 Prescott Place, London SW4 6BS. Tel: 071 720 8055.

Myasthenia Gravis Association, Central Office, Keynes House, 77 Nottingham Road, Derby DE1 3QS. Tel: 0332 290219.

National Association for Colitis and Crohn's Disease, 98A London Rd, St Albans, Herts. AL1 1NX. Tel: 0727 844296.

National Asthma Campaign, Providence House, Providence Place, London. NW5 2LX. Tel: 071 267 1361.

National Autistic Society, 276 Willesden Lane, London NW2 5RB. Tel: 081 451 1114.

National Back Pain Association, 16 Elmtree Road, Teddington, Middx TW11 8ST. Tel: 081 977 5474.

National Childbirth Trust, Alexandra House, Oldham Terrace, Acton, London W3 6NH. Tel: 081 992 8637.

National Childrens Bureau, 8 Wakely Street, London. EC1V Tel: 071 278 9441.

National Council for One Parent Families, 255 Kentish Town Road, London. NW5 2LX. Tel: 071 267 1361.

National Council for Vocational Qualifications, 222 Euston Road, London NW1 2BZ. Tel: 071 387 9898.

National Deaf-Blind and Rubella Association (SENSE), 11-13 Clifton Terrace, London N4. Tel: 071 278 1005.

National Deaf Blind League, 18 Rainbow Court, Paston Ridings, Peterborough PE4 6UP. Tel: 0733 73511.

National Meningitis Trust, Fern House, Bath Road, Stroud, Glos GL5 3TJ. Tel: 0453 751 738. Helpline 0453 755 049.

National Osteoporosis Society, PO Box 10, Radstock, Bath. BA3 3YB. Tel: 0761 432 472.

National Schizophrenia Fellowship, 28 Castle Street, Kingston-upon-Thames, Surrey KT1 1SS. Tel: 081 547 3937.

National Society for Epilepsy, Information Department, Chalfont St Peter, Buckinghamshire SL9 0RJ. Tel: 0494 873991.

National Society for the Prevention of Cruelty to Children (NSPCC), 67 Saffron Hill, London, EC1N 8RS. Tel: 071 242 1626.

National Toy Libraries Association, 68 Churchway, London NW1 1LT. 071 387 9592.

Nottingham Rehab Ltd, 17 Ludlow Hill Road, Melton Road, West Bridgford, Nottingham NG2 6HD. Tel: 0602 452345. Activity materials and aids – catalogue available.

Open College, St Paul's, 781 Wilmslow Rd, Didsbury, Greater Manchester M20 8RW. Tel: 061 434 0007.

Open University, Information Office, Department of Health and Social Welfare, Milton Keynes MK7 6AA. Tel: 0908 653743.

Paget's Disease, (National Association for the Relief of), Room B304, CSB Hope Hospital, Salford, Manchester. M6 8HD. Tel: 061 787 4949.

Pain Society, 9 Bedford Square, London WC1B 3RA. Tel: 071 631 1650.

Parkinson's Disease Society of the UK, 22 Upper Woburn Place, London WC1H 0RA. Tel: 071 383 3513.

Patients Association, 18 Victoria Park Square, Bethnal Green, London E2 9PF. Tel: 081 981 5676/5695.

Pavilion Publishing (Brighton) Ltd, 42 Lansdowne Place Hove, East Sussex. Tel: 0273 623222. Training materials.

Perthes Disease Association, 42 Woodland

Road, Guildford, Surrey GU1 1RW. Tel: 0483 306637.

PHAB (Physically Handicapped and Able-Bodied together) 14 London Rd, Croydon CR0 2TA. Tel: 081 667 9443.

Phenylketonuria (National Society for), 7 Southfield Close, Willem, Milton Keynes MK15 9LL. Tel: 0908 691653.

Positively Women, 5 Sebastian St, London, EC1V 0HE Tel. 071 490 5515

Pre-school Play Groups Association, 61-63 Kings Cross Road London WC1X 9LL. Tel: 071 833 0991.

Psoriasis Association (PA), 7, Milton Street, Northampton NN2 7JG. Tel: 0604 711129.

QUIT (help to stop smoking), Victory House, 170, Tottenham Court Rd, London W1P 0HA. Tel: 071 388 5775. Quitline 071 487 3000.

Royal College of Nursing of the UK, 20 Cavendish Square, London W1M 0AB. Tel: 071 409 3333.

Royal National Institute for the Blind, 224 Great Portland Street, London W1N 6AA. Tel: 071 388 1266.

Royal National Institute for the Deaf, 105 Gower Street, London WC1E 6AH. Tel: 071 387 8033.

Royal Society for the Prevention of Accidents, Cannon House, The Priory, Queensway, Birmingham. B4 6BS. Tel: 021 200 2461.

Samaritans, 10, The Grove, Slough, Berkshire. SL1 1QP. Tel: 0753 532713.

Sickle Cell and Thalassaemia Information Centre, St Leonard's Hospital, Nutall St, London N1 5LZ. Tel: 071 739 8484.

Sickle Cell Society, 54, Station Road, London. NW10 4UA. Tel: 081 961 7795

Social Care Association, 23a Victoria Rd, Surbiton, Surrey. Tel: 081 390 6831/4639.

Schizophrenia Association of Great Britain. Bryn Hyfryd, The Crescent, Bangor, Gwynedd LL57 2AG. Tel: 0248 354048.

SCOPE (formally the Spastics Society), 12 Park Crescent, London W1N 4EQ. Tel: 071 636 5020.

Spinal Injuries Association, Newpoint House, 76 St James's Lane, London N10 3DF. Tel: 081 444 2121. Helpline 081 883 4296.

SPOD (Sexual and personal relationships of disabled people) 286 Camden Rd, London N7 0BJ. Tel: 071 607 8851.

Stillbirth and Neonatal Death Society (SANDS) 28 Portland Place London W1N 4DE. Tel: 071 436 5881.

St John Ambulance, 1 Grosvenor Cresent, London. SW1X 7EF. Tel: 071 235 5231.

Stroke Association, CHSA House 123-127, Whitecross Street, London. EC1Y 8JJ. Tel: 071 490 7999.

Talking Books for the Handicapped (National Listening Library), 12 Lant Street, London SE1 1QR. Tel: 071 407 9417. A postal lending library service of literature recorded on long-playing cassettes.

Terence Higgins Trust, 52,54 Grays Inn Road. London, WC1X 8JU. Tel: 071 831 0330.

TFH, 76 Barracks Road, Sandy Lane Industrial Estate, Stourport-on-Severn, Worcestershire DY13 9QB. Tel: 0299 827820. Games, puzzles, pastimes etc for disabled/older people.

Turner Syndrome Society, Child Growth Foundation, 2 Mayfield Avenue, London W4 1PW. Tel: 081 994 7625.

United Kingdom Central Council For Nursing, Midwifery and Health Visiting, 23 Portland Place, London. W1N 3AF. Tel: 071 637 7181.

UK Thalassaemia Society, 107 Nightingale Lane London. N8 7QY. Tel: 081 348 0437

University of the Third Age, 1 Stockwell Green, SW9 9JF. Tel: 071 737 2541. Promotes and organises self-help educational activities for older people.

Urostomy Association, Buckland, Beaumont Park, Danbury, Essex. CM3 4DE. Tel: 0245 224294.

Victim Support, Cranmer House, 39 Brixton road, London SW9 6DZ. Tel: 071 735 9166.

Winslow Press, Telford Road, Bicester, Oxfordshire OX6 0TS. Tel: 0869 244733.

Glossary of terms

Abuse. Physical, verbal or emotional mistreatment or exploitation of another person against their best interests.

Accreditation of Prior Learning (for NVQ). The assessment of an individual's past achievements against national standards.

Acute. Used to describe an illness or condition that is of relatively short duration, and usually severe.

Adrenaline. A naturally occurring hormone, a synthetic version of which can be given by injection in the event of a respiratory or cardiac arrest. It dilates the air tubes and stimulates the heart to beat faster. It also stimulates the liver to release stored sugar.

Advocate. A person who supports, encourages, defends and negotiates on behalf of another by representing them where they are unsure or unable to represent themselves.

Agitation. An extreme state of upset where the person may experience physical signs of restlessness and feel uneasy and tense.

AIDS (Acquired Immunodeficiency Syndrome – see also HIV). A condition caused by a virus called Human Immunodeficiency Virus (HIV). It damages the defence system so that the body cannot fight infection. AIDS can cause people to develop certain forms of cancer, and to get serious infections of the lungs, digestive system, the brain and skin. It is passed on by exchanging body fluids such as blood, semen and vaginal fluids.

Allergy. A reaction to a substance to which a person is sensitive. Examples include fur, dust, alcohol, certain foods, insect stings and medicines. Usually causes skin rashes, but can be more severe causing difficulty with breathing due to swelling of the throat and airway. Death can occur. (See also Anaphylaxis).

Alzheimer's disease (see also Dementia). A form of dementia characterised by changes to the brain, although the particular cause is unknown. Disorientation, loss of memory, and intellectual function, apathy and difficulty with coordinating movement, speech and thoughts, and disorientation, are common features.

Amnesia. Loss of memory.

Anaemia. Shortage of the oxygen-carrying part (haemoglobin) of the blood's red cells. This may be because the body is losing too much haemoglobin (eg due to bleeding) or because it is not making enough (eg due to a shortage of iron in the diet).

Anaesthetic. A substance that can cause temporary loss of the sensation of pain or consciousness. As a "local" anaesthetic it numbs a specific part of the body only. As a "general" anaesthetic it causes the patient to lose consciousness.

Analgesics. Medicines that provide relief from pain.

Anaphylactic shock. A severe reaction causing swelling of the airway and possible respiratory and cardiac arrest. It can occur when a medicine or injection is given. It can also occur if people are allergic to a particular food or are bitten or stung by an insect.

Angina. Chest pain due to oxygen shortage in the heart muscles. Caused by narrowing or blockage of the coronary arteries which supply the heart muscle with oxygen.

Anorexia. This is the loss of desire to eat. Emotional disturbances, such as depression, may induce a chronic state of anorexia.

Antibiotics. Medicines which either kill bacteria or stop them multiplying. They have no effect on a virus.

Anticonvulsant drugs. Medicines which are used to treat epilepsy.

Anti-depressant drugs. Medicines that are used in the treatment of depression. These drugs act upon and stimulate parts of the nervous system.

Anti-emetics. Medicines that are used to prevent nausea and sickness.

Anti-histamine. Medicines and creams used to counter the symptoms of an allergic reaction, eg irritation and itching of the skin.

Anus (see also Colon and Rectum). The muscular ring at the end of the intestinal canal.

Anxiety state. A condition in which the individual is so worried about a certain situation, that their life is severely restricted. The main characteristic is the inability to relax.

Arteriosclerosis. A gradual loss of elasticity in the walls of arteries due to thickening and the build up of calcium and cholesterol deposits. This may cause decreased blood flow and oxygen supply to essential parts of the brain and body.

Artery. A blood vessel carrying blood containing oxygen around the body.

Arthritis (see also Osteoarthritis and Rheumatoid Arthritis). Inflammation causing pain, stiffness or swelling in one or more joints. There may be serious deformity, (eg of the hands) and disability. There are several different types including osteoarthritis and rheumatoid arthritis. Main causes are inflammation, and the effects of wear and tear.

Aseptic. Free from germs and bacteria that cause infection.

Assessment. The systematic collection of information by observing, interviewing and examining an individual and their social environment in order to develop a plan of care.

Assessment (for NVQ). The process of collecting evidence and making judgements on whether national standards have been met.

Assessment centre (for NVQ). A consortium or single organisation which has had its assessment arrangements approved by an awarding body.

Assessment methods (for NVQ). Naturalistic observation and other methods used to assess candidate competence.

Assessors (for NVQ). Individuals approved by assessment centres to judge evidence of competence.

Asthma. A condition in which the tubes of the lung have a fluctuating and reversible tendency to narrow causing breathlessness, coughing, wheezing or chest tightness. It may be triggered by an allergy.

Audiometer. A machine used to test a person's ability to hear normally.

Audit (see also Standards and Quality Assurance). A methodical process of examining (for example, practical care, record keeping and client satisfaction with services) against agreed standards.

Autopsy. See post mortem.

Awards in care A set of 20 NVQs at Level 2 and 3 with wide availability across health and social care.

Barrier cream. A cream, usually water based, that is applied to the skin to prevent drying or damage where for example a person may be incontinent.

BCG. A vaccine given to prevent people contracting Tuberculosis (TB). See also Immunisation.

Benign. When describing a tumour means favourable, non-cancerous, usually contained within a capsule and not spreading to other parts of the body.

Bereavement. The human response to loss, usually as a result of a person dying. It also occurs when a person has lost something personal and important to them, such as their home, or a limb.

Blood pressure. The force of blood in the arteries measured in millimetres of mercury by a machine called a sphygmo-manometer. Blood pressures are written down as two figures. The top figure is called "systolic" and the bottom figure is called "diastolic". How high or low the blood pressure is depends on the strength of the heart beat and the condition of the arteries.

Bradycardia. A marked slowing of the rate of the heart.

Braille. A system of writing and printing by means of raised points representing letters which allows blind and partially sighted people to read by touch.

Bronchitis. Inflammation of the air tubes of the lungs. It may be "acute" due to infection, or "chronic" due to excessive production of mucus caused by many factors including pollution and smoking.

Bronchodilators. Medicines used to widen the lung airways.

Cancer. A large group of diseases which are linked together. In each case there is uncontrolled new abnormal tissue growth of the affected part/s of the body. The outlook for each cancer sufferer is dependent upon the site and type of the growth.

Capillaries. Tiny blood vessels that lie between arteries bringing blood to the tissues, and veins taking blood away.

Cardiac arrest. Used to describe a situation in which the heart suddenly stops beating.

Cardio-pulmonary resuscitation (CPR). The technique used to try and restart a heart after a person has had a cardiac arrest. It includes breathing into the person's lungs and externally massaging the heart in a regular and systematic way.

Care manager. A person who is responsible for coordinating an individual's assessment and package of care through a variety of agencies.

Care package. The term used to describe a plan of care where more than one agency is involved. It may include health services, social services, independent and voluntary workers as well as family carers.

Carer. The term usually applied to a person who provides care at home without receiving a salary or wage. Most often it is a female relative of a dependent person.

Cataract. A clouding of the lens of the eye preventing light passing through it. Vision becomes very dim or is lost altogether.

Catheter. A tube which is passed into the body to drain away fluids. The most common is the urinary catheter for draining the bladder.

Cerebral palsy. Permanent and usually non-progressive damage to the brain before, during or soon after birth. Mental impairment may take place. There is usually some loss of the use of limbs.

Cerebrovascular accident (CVA). See Stroke.

Cervix. The neck of the womb.

Chemotherapy. The treatment of disease by medicines or chemicals. The term is often used for cancer treatment, which can make the person feel very unwell, nauseous and cause hair loss.

Child Health Surveillance. The term used to describe a system used nationally to monitor the growth and development of children. It includes measuring weight, height, and ensuring that children can carry out activities appropriate to their age.

Chronic. A term used to describe a long standing and continued disease process. There may be progressive deterioration (sometimes despite treatment).

Circumcision. An operation to remove all or part of the foreskin of the penis.

Cleft palate. A defect in the roof of the mouth causing impaired speech. Usually occurs before a child is born. It can be treated successfully with surgery.

Cognition. Consciously knowing, understanding and having insight into personal and environmental events. The person may not necessarily be able to take action.

Colic. A sharp pain resulting from spasm of a muscle, commonly the stomach and gut.

Colon (see also Anus and Rectum). A part of the large intestine that absorbs nutrients and fluid from the diet. It ends at the anus.

Colostomy. See Stoma.

Community psychiatric nurse. A qualified mental health nurse who works with people living in their own homes or attending mental health centres.

Competence (for NVQ). The ability to perform an activity to the agreed standard. The assessment of competence forms the basis for NVQs and SVQs.

Compliance aid. A storage box for tablets. Contains sections for each day and the time that the medicine should be taken. Helps to remind people of when to take medicines.

Compress. Soft pad of gauze or cloth used to apply heat, cold or medications to the surface of the body.

Concussion. A temporary loss of consciousness due to a knock on the head. The person becomes pale, has a feeble pulse and shallow breathing.

Confusion. Conditions in which consciousness is clouded, so that the individual is unable to think clearly or act rationally. Confusional states may be temporary, due to acute illness (toxic confusional states), or long term and irreversible.

Connective tissue. The supporting tissues of the body, found under the skin, between muscles, and supporting blood vessels and nerves. Their functions are mainly mechanical, connecting other active tissues and organs.

Constipation. Incomplete or infrequent action of the bowels, due to lack of muscle activity, insufficient fluids or inadequate diet.

Continence (see also Incontinence). The ability to control the functions of passing urine or faeces when desired.

Contra-indication. A reason for not doing something, such as giving a medicine as this could have an adverse affect on the person.

Coronary artery disease. Narrowing or blockage of the arteries supplying the heart with oxygen. Usually due to blockage of the coronary arteries. Also known as coronary heart disease or coronary vascular disease.

Counselling. A skilled method of listening to and talking with a person or a group of people, to enable them to overcome a problem, make a decision or accept their circumstances.

Cramp. Painful contraction of a muscle, associated with salt loss. Failure to replace salt or fluids, a lack of oxygen reaching the muscle, or poisons of various kinds may be the cause.

Culture. The values, attitudes, lifestyle and customs shared by a group of people and passed from one generation to the next.

Cyanosed. Bluish discolouration of the skin, particularly the lips, due to shortage of oxygen supply.

Cystic fibrosis. An inherited disorder causing glands to produce abnormally thick secretions, particularly in the lungs, pancreas and sweat glands. It is diagnosed by analysing sweat for high levels of body salts such as sodium and chloride. It is treated by exercises to drain the lungs, careful attention to diet and preventing infections.

Cytology. The microscopic study of the cells of the body.

Defaecation. The act of opening the bowels.

Dehydration. Excessive loss of fluid from the body caused by vomiting, diarrhoea or sweating or because of inadequate fluid intake.

Dementia (see also Alzheimer's disease). An organic mental illness caused by changes to the brain. This may be a result of disease or damage. The principal changes include inability to learn and retain information, inability to recall recent events, and feelings of anxiety and depression. This leads to disorientation and confused behaviour.

Depression. A profound sadness, distinct from normal bereavement or loss. Its features include reduced enjoyment, slowness and a lack of interest in life or the lives of others.

Dexterity. The ability to use fingers and hands to undertake everyday activities.

Diabetes. Failure of the pancreas in the body to produce insulin, or failure of the body to use the insulin correctly. Insulin breaks down sugary foods, allowing the body to use it for energy. Diabetes results in too much sugar circulating in the blood. Normal body functioning, for example wound healing, is affected by the condition. It is treated by diet alone, medicines or insulin.

Digoxin. One of the earliest discovered medicines which was found to have a beneficial effect on the failing heart.

Disorientation. A state of confusion in which an individual has lost a sense of where they are, what time it is and what they are doing.

District nurse. A registered nurse who has also undertaken a one year university course in order to provide specialist nursing care and advice to people living at home. The district nurse provides services in family doctor surgeries.

Diuretic. A medicine which stimulates the kidney to produce more urine.

Diverticulitis. A condition in which there is inflammation of small pockets (diverticulae) of large bowel which stick through the muscle surrounding the bowel at weak points. Generally caused by long-standing constipation.

Down's syndrome. A congenital disorder caused by an extra chromosome. The person may have marked learning difficulties and heart problems.

Dysarthria. A speech disorder caused by poor muscle movement or poor muscle co-ordination, often following a stroke.

Dyslexia. Difficulty with reading and writing.

Dysphagia. Difficulty with swallowing.

Dysphasia. A language disorder which may affect understanding, speaking, reading and writing (often due to a stroke).

Eczema. A condition of the skin causing dryness, flaking and extreme itching.

Elimination. The removal of waste matter from the body.

Empowerment. Giving an individual permission, support and power to enable them to control what is happening to them.

Encephalitis. Inflammation of the brain, ususally due to a virus.

Enema. Procedure involving the introduction of a fluid into the rectum for cleansing or therapeutic purposes.

Enteral feeding. Provision of nutrients through a tube directly into the stomach when the person cannot chew or swallow food but can digest and absorb the nutrients.

Enuresis (nocturnal). Bed wetting.

Epilepsy. A condition in which excessive or unregulated electrical activity in the brain causes fits. These may involve the whole body with loss of consciousness –

"grand mal" – or parts of the body, involving perhaps a short loss of full consciousness, known as "petit mal" fits. "Focal fits" are said to occur when only one part of the body, arms or legs, is affected.

Ethnicity (see also Culture). A group's sense of identity associated with race, heritage, upbringing and values.

Evidence (for NVQ). Proof in support of the judgement made by an assessor that a candidate is competent.

Exertion. The amount of effort a person puts into carrying out a task. This may be physical, in walking or getting out of bed. It can also be mental, for example struggling to remember recent events.

Faeces. Waste matter which is indigestible such as fibre, excreted by the bowel.

Fainting. A temporary loss of consciousness due to a fall in blood pressure. The person usually falls to the floor, as this is the way in which the body attempts to restore the blood circulation, so that oxygen can reach the brain.

Fatigue. State of extreme exhaustion or loss of strength.

Fibre (in diet). Used to describe food that is high in roughage, indigestible, and stimulates the action of the intestine (bowel).

Flatulence. Excessive wind, usually causing discomfort and pain.

Fluoride. A salt added to drinking water and toothpaste to prevent tooth decay. Fluoride drops can also be given to children in the early years.

Formula milk. A powdered milk given to babies and young children that contains all the essential nutrients and attempts to match breast milk.

Fracture. A broken bone. The signs and symptoms include pain, swelling, loss of power and shortening of the affected limb.

Gangrene. Death of body tissue usually due to loss of blood supply.

Gender. Relating to the male or female sex.

Genital. Relates to the sexual organs of the man or woman.

Glaucoma. An illness in which abnormally high fluid pressure inside the eye can cause permanent damage.

Guardian. A person who assigns themselves or is appointed legally to look after and take responsibility for another.

Guarding. A defensive action that a person may take to safeguard themselves or to prevent any pain. It may include not wishing to talk about difficult subjects or holding oneself in a comfortable position that prevents physical pain.

Haemorrhoids. Piles.

Health education. Educational activities directed towards enhancing or maintaining the health and wellbeing of others.

Health visitor. A registered nurse who has also undertaken a one year university course in order to provide specialist care and advice on how to stay healthy. The health visitor works with all age groups and may provide services in family doctor surgeries.

Heart attack. Damage to an area of the heart muscle due to obstruction of the artery supplying this area with blood. Usually preceded by extreme chest pain.

Heart failure. The failure by the heart to pump blood around the body efficiently. The most common symptoms are breathlessness, tiredness and swollen ankles.

Hemiplegia. Paralysis of one side of the body. Usually caused by stroke or as a result of injury or disease to the brain.

Hernia. Protrusion of an organ from its normal position in the body into another. The most common is the inguinal hernia in which bowel pushes through defects in the muscle of the groin. Also known as a "rupture".

HIV (Human Immunodeficiency Virus). The virus that causes AIDS. It is not one virus, but a family of many similar viruses. It weakens the body's defence system by entering and destroying white cells that normally protect our body from infection.

Hydrocephalus. Accumulation of fluid in and around the brain.

Hypertension (see also Blood pressure). A condition in which the blood pressure is higher than it should be for an individual person. Blood pressures are written down as two figures. The top figure is called the "systolic" and the bottom figure is known as the "diastolic".

Hypotension. A condition in which the blood pressure is lower than it should be.

Hypothermia. Body temperature below the usual value of 37 degrees centigrade. At about 35 degrees centigrade confusion and listlessness may begin. Below 33 degrees centigrade the breathing and pulse rate and blood pressure may start to fall. If prolonged, death may occur.

Ileostomy (see Stoma).

Immunisation. The process by which a small safe dose of an infectious disease is given to build up body immune resistance.

Impairment. A reduction or weakening of any body function.

Incontinence (see also Continence). The inability to control the passage of urine or faeces until a suitable time and place is found. Urinary incontinence may occur when abdominal pressure, through coughing or lifting heavy weights, causes urine to leak from the bladder and urethra. Faecal incontinence is caused by a loss of control of the anus. Disorientation may also cause incontinence.

Infarct. An area of the body which is damaged or dies as a result of not receiving enough oxygen from its arteries. This supply failure is usually due to a blockage of or haemorrhage from the artery. Frequently used as "coronary" or "myocardial" infarct to describe the damage done to heart muscle after a heart attack.

Infusion. Introduction of a substance, such as a medicine in fluid form, directly into a vein or under the skin. May be attached to a mechanical pump to ensure that the correct amount is given over a period of time.

Insomnia. Difficulty getting to sleep or staying asleep for a long time.

Intestine. The bowel.

Intractable. Commonly used in reference to pain, that

is difficult to control or cure.

Key worker. Every client is assigned a key worker, to deal with their case, and to instruct other care assistants in any special treatments, preferences etc.

Larynx. The voice organ. Vocal cords of elastic tissue are spread across it. The vibrations and contractions of these produce the changes in the pitch of the voice.

Laxative. A medicine to encourage passing faeces.

Legislation. Acts of Parliament passed by the Government that must be upheld under the law.

Local authority. A body responsible for a range of public services, such as housing and recreation provided in a given area, usually a geographical Borough or Council.

Malabsorption. The failure of the gut to absorb nutrients and food. It can lead to malnutrition.

Malignant. A type of tumour that spreads and grows uncontrollably.

Malnutrition (see also nutrition). Under-nourishment due to poor diet or disease that prevents absorption of essential nutrients.

Manometer. A device for measuring the pressure of a fluid.

Medication (see also Sedation and Tranquilliser). Used to describe tablets, liquids or injections used with the aim of improving a person's physical or mental condition.

Melaena. The production of black, tarry stools containing blood from the upper part of the gut.

Meningitis. A serious infection of the tissues surrounding the brain.

Metabolism. The sum total of the chemical processes that occur in living organisms, resulting in growth, production of energy, elimination of waste material.

Micturition. The act of emptying the bladder of urine.

Monitored drug dosage system. A system of providing medicines that are dispensed and sealed by the pharmacist in weekly or monthly packs.

Motor neurone disease. A disease in which there is progressive destruction of some of the nerves responsible for stimulating muscles. This causes weakness and problems with movement, breathing and swallowing. The cause is unknown.

Motor strength. The strength of the muscle which stimulates the limbs and body to move.

Mucous membrane. A mucus-secreting membrane that lines body cavities (eg lungs) or passages that are open to the external environment (eg mouth, nose, vagina).

Mucus. The slimy protective secretion of the mucus membranes.

Multiple sclerosis. An often fluctuating, sometimes progressive disease of the brain and spinal cord in which plaques replace normal nerve tissue. This can cause a range of symptoms, including difficulty with coordinating movement, incontinence and problems with vision and speech.

Muscular dystrophy. A group of muscle disorders which are usually passed on through families and become apparent in childhood and adolescence.

Named nurse. An initiative within the UK to ensure that all people receiving nursing care have a "named nurse" that they can directly relate to.

Nausea. The sensation of feeling sick.

Nebuliser. Equipment that adds drops of water or medicine to compressed air or oxygen so that it can be absorbed more effectively or dislodge mucus in the air passages and lungs.

Neurological. Relating to the body's brain and nerves.

Neuro-transmitters. Chemical substances that help to pass a signal down a nerve.

Nutrition. The intake of nutrients (in food and drink) and their assimilation into body tissue.

National Council for Vocational Qualifications (NCVQ). Sets out the structure and framework of vocational qualifications for England, Wales and Northern Ireland. (SCOTVEC is the equivalent for Scotland.)

NVQs – National Vocational Qualifications. Practical work-based qualifications. See chapter 24.

Occupational therapist. A health care practitioner who is qualified to diagnose and teach people with an illness or disability to use aids and adaptations for everyday living and working.

Oedema. Excess tissue fluid, often around ankles, at the base of the spine or in the heart and lungs.

Orthoptist. A specialist practitioner who is trained to diagnose and treat eye conditions such as a squint.

Osteoarthritis (see also Arthritis & Rheumatoid arthritis). A form of arthritis occurring in the joints of older people. It is usually very painful. There is destruction of the spongy pads between bones, and small bony growths at the edges of the bone joint.

Paediatrics. A branch of medicine specialising in babies and children.

Palliative. Treatment that relieves or reduces uncomfortable symptoms, such as pain, but does not provide a cure.

Paralysis. Loss of movement (but not sensation) in a muscle or group of muscles normally under the person's control. May be due to damage to the muscle itself or to its nerve supply.

Parent Held Records. Health records used by health visitors that record details of a child's development and family health. It is kept by the parent or guardian rather than by a health professional.

Parkinsonism. Symptoms such as shaking or trembling, rhythmical muscular tremors, rigidity and a mask-like face that shows no emotion. Thumb and fore fingers may move in a "rolling" fashion. It can be caused by tranquillisers.

Peak flow. The measurement of air as it is expelled from the lungs.

Performance criteria (for NVQ). A set of outcomes related to an element of performance by which an assessor can judge that a candidate can work to the required standard.

Personality. The mental make-up of a person. The way that they respond is influenced by life events and experiences, and their attitudes to situations.

Pharmacist. Practitioner trained to make up prescribed medicines and provide advice and information on side effects and contra-indications.

Photophobia. Intolerance to light.

Physiotherapist. A health care practitioner who is qualified to diagnose, teach and apply therapies, usually involving muscles and bones, to people who are ill, have an injury or disability, in order to restore them to health.

Pneumonia. Inflammation of the lungs due to bacterial, viral or fungal infections.

Podiatrist. Practitioner trained to diagnose and treat disorders of the feet.

Prescription. A legal document that must be used and signed by a doctor for issuing medicines. It must contain the name, dose and frequency of the medicines.

Pressure sore. An area of skin and underlying tissues which dies as a result of pressure persistently preventing the flow of blood through its blood vessels. It can cause an ulcer or sore to develop, particularly if the skin is broken.

Prognosis. The outlook for a person with a disease, in terms of disability and death.

Prostate. A gland at the base of the bladder in men. It may become enlarged due to disease or old age, causing difficulty in passing urine.

Prosthesis. Manufactured substitute for a part of the body (for example an artificial leg, false teeth, breast).

Pruritus. Itching.

Pulse. The regular expansion and contraction of an artery produced by waves of pressure as blood is pumped from the heart.

Pyrexia. Raised body temperature.

Quality Assurance (see also Audit and Standard). A system of evaluating and auditing the standards of a service to ensure that the best possible service is provided in terms of value for money and client satisfaction.

Racism. Discrimination against a person on the grounds of skin colour and/or ethnic origin.

Range statements (for NVQ). The breadth of contexts in which a candidate is expected to demonstrate competence (linked to an element of competence).

Reality orientation. The way in which older people with mental illness are helped to keep in touch with the world around them. This may be through the use of large clocks, signs on doors, and newspapers.

Recovery position. The safest position in which to place a person who is unconscious. The purpose is to ensure that the mouth is kept open to allow breathing and to permit saliva, vomit or blood to flow out rather than going into the lungs. Movement should be minimal, rolling the person onto their left side where possible. If a back injury is suspected, the person should only be moved as a life-saving measure.

Rectum (see also Colon). The lower end of the bowel leading out to the anus.

Rehabilitation. The process by which a team of workers restores a person who has had a serious illness or injury to as near as possible their previous state of health.

Reminiscence therapy. Active participation by individuals or groups, using past life events to understand the reasons for their mental health problems. The past can also be used as a basis to share concerns and anxieties, since people with dementia are more likely to

have a better memory for long term events than for more recent events.

Respiratory arrest. Used to describe a situation in which a person stops breathing, but before the heart stops beating. There can be more than one cause.

Respite. Temporary relief services for the main carer of a dependent person in the home or other setting.

Rheumatism. The term is loosely applied to any pain of unknown cause in the joints or muscles. Small swellings may appear under the skin, particularly around bony ridges. There may be fever, sweating and pain and stiffness in the joints.

Rheumatoid arthritis (see also Arthritis and Osteoarthritis). Arthritis occurring in the small and large joints of people of all ages. The cause is unknown.

Role reversal. A situation in which a person exchanges a pattern of behaviour with another. For example a daughter may have to take on a mothering role to her own mother if she requires care.

Sacrum. Part of the lower end of the spine.

School nurse. A registered nurse, usually with a specific qualification to provide care and health assessments for children of school age.

Sedative (see also Medication and Tranquilliser). Having a calming or soothing effect.

Sexuality. A part of the human personality that relates in physical, emotional and social dimensions to the way a person identifies and values themself. It includes their gender, appearance and sexual preferences.

Sharps. Any piece of equipment used that could cause injury by stabbing or cutting a person if not disposed of safely.

Shock. This may arise out of fear or pain, it may also be the result of loss of blood, as a reaction to medicines, or contact with electrical currents. It is the condition in which there is a sudden fall in blood pressure, which if untreated will lead to a lack of oxygen in the tissues.

Sickle cell anaemia. A severe, chronic, incurable disease of the blood. The red blood cell adopts a crescent shape and becomes fragile. This results in a decrease of oxygen being supplied to body organs and tissues causing acute and long term problems. More common in black and ethnic minority individuals.

Social services. A department of the local authority that employs social care workers to enable people to live independently at home by providing practical help and advice. Examples include social workers, welfare rights officers, disablement officers and care assistants.

Social worker. A professional trained to counsel clients and families, helping them seek community and financial resources to enable them to live independently in the community or other setting.

Specific gravity. The density of a fluid compared to an equal volume of water. Often used to measure urine to detect for example kidney disease.

Sphincter. A muscular ring which surrounds the opening of a hollow organ, such as the bladder. It controls the escape of the content of the organ until a suitable time.

Spina bifida. A congenital disease in which there is a defect in the bones of the spine. It can be mild and cause no symptoms. In more serious forms the spinal cord can be damaged causing paralysis of the legs, and incontinence of urine and faeces, often accompanied by hydrocephalus and mental retardation.

Sprain. An injury to a ligament when the joint it is supporting is forced through a range of movements greater than normal, without dislocation or fracture.

Sputum. Excess secretion from the lungs that contains mucus and saliva. It may also contain bacteria.

Squint. A fixed deviation of the eye from its normal direction. Called "convergent" when the eye turns towards the nose and "divergent" when it turns away from the nose.

Standard. A guide that serves as a basis for measuring how good or bad a particular service or practice is. (See also Audit and Quality Assurance.)

Stereotype. A commonly held belief about a behaviour, individual or group that is not always true.

Stethoscope. A device for listening to sounds within the body, such as heart beat, bowel sounds and breathing, that cannot otherwise be heard by the human ear.

Stoma. A surgical procedure in which an opening is made on the abdominal wall to allow the passage of intestinal contents (colostomy and ileostomy) or urine (urostomy) from the bladder.

Stool. A word used to describe faeces.

Stress. Stress reactions, both physical and mental, occur when the individual is unable to cope with all the demands made upon them. If extreme, it may be called "burn-out".

Stroke (see also Cerebrovascular accident). A rapid brain disorder usually caused by a blockage in or haemorrhage from one of the main arteries of the brain. Speech and movement are commonly affected. Other functions may be damaged depending upon which artery is affected. Recovery depends on the extent of the damage.

Subcutaneous. Relates to an injection or infusion given into the skin tissue at a 45 degree angle, rather than into the muscle (intramuscular).

Syringe driver. A battery-driven device for giving drugs (usually pain killers) over a period of time via a subcutaneous needle under the skin.

Systole. The maximum level of blood pressure measured between heart contractions.

Tachycardia. A marked increase in heart rate.

Thalassaemia. An inherited type of anaemia caused by deficient red blood cells. Frequent transfusions are required to maintain the oxygen carrying capacity of the blood. People of Mediterranean origin are more often affected than others.

Therapy. The science and art of treating people. Therapy may be in the form of medicine and surgery, but also involves personal approaches, such as counselling or providing the right environment in which a person feels comfortable and safe.

Thrombosis. The formation of a blood clot on the lining of an artery or vein which may partially or completely block the blood flow through it.

Thrush. A fungal infection usually affecting the mucous membranes such as the mouth and vagina.

Toxin. Any poisonous compound. It may be caused by bacteria multiplying in the body.

Tracheostomy. A temporary or permanent surgical opening above the Adam's apple. It allows a person to breathe when the throat or upper airway is diseased or damaged.

Tranquilliser (see also Medication and Sedation). Medicines that allay anxiety and have a calming effect on the person. They may also prevent them from feeling pain.

Trauma. A wound or injury, physical or emotional. Emotional trauma can be a cause of mental illness.

Tumour. A lump or swelling in the body that is not inflamed. A benign tumour does not grow in other parts of the body. A malignant tumour may spread to other organs.

Ulcer. An erosion and inflammation of the skin or mucous membranes. Examples include venous leg ulcers, caused by poor skin condition and poor return of blood to the heart. Arterial leg ulcers are caused by poor blood supply.

Universal precautions. The wearing of gloves, protective clothing and correct cleaning and disposal of waste to prevent the spread of infection from blood and body fluids.

Ureters. The tubes which drain urine from the kidneys into the bladder.

Urethra. The tube that carries urine from the bladder to outside the body.

Urine. Waste products in liquid form that are produced in the kidney and emptied from the body via the bladder.

Urinary tract infection. An infection that affects the bladder or the urethra. It may result in the person wanting to pass urine frequently, cause pain and a stinging sensation.

Urostomy. See Stoma.

Value base unit (for NVQ). This is the "O" Unit which embeds in NVQ awards in care the principles of good practice: anti-discrimination, confidentiality, rights and choice, respect for beliefs and identity and effective communication.

Varicose veins. A condition, usually of the lower leg, in which the veins are swollen and may be twisted due to structural changes in the walls or valves of the vessels. These veins have difficulty returning blood back to the heart. Knocks to varicose veins commonly cause leg ulcers in older people.

Vascular. Relating to blood vessels, usually arteries or veins.

Vein. A vessel carrying blood from the capillaries back to the heart after oxygen has been removed by the tissues and organs that need it.

Vertigo. A feeling of dizziness accompanied by a feeling that either oneself or one's surroundings are spinning.

Visual acuity. A measurement of how much a person can see at a particular distance, usually six metres, to identify whether they are short- or long-sighted.

Index